MW01289059

They call ME a QUACK!

They call ME a QUACK!

My personal journey from traditional to alternative medicine

W. Gene Schroeder, M.D., H.M.D.

iUniverse, Inc.

New York Lincoln Shanghai

They call ME a QUACK!
My personal journey from traditional to alternative medicine

All Rights Reserved © 2004 by W. Gene Schroeder, M.D., H.M.D.

No part of this book may be reproduced or transmitted in any form or by any means, graphic, electronic, or mechanical, including photocopying, recording, taping, or by any information storage retrieval system, without the written permission of the publisher.

iUniverse, Inc.

For information address:
iUniverse, Inc.
2021 Pine Lake Road, Suite 100
Lincoln, NE 68512
www.iuniverse.com

The suggestions in this book are not meant to be a substitute for a careful medical evaluation by your doctor. This book is intended for educational purposes and the use of the information presented should be used with discretion.

ISBN: 0-595-32580-7

Printed in the United States of America

Dedication

I wish to dedicate this book to my wonderful patients and beautiful loving wife, Kathleen. My journey as both a physician and author was made possible only by the input, devotion, cooperation and respect of my patients. Kathleen has given me constant understanding, encouragement, support and love. I have been truly blessed with life's greatest offerings—people who love me.

To date I have been able to weather the many problems that traditional medicine has fostered in my life. I believe that persistence and perseverance have enabled me to be a better and more effective physician, one who has shown and will continue to show others the advantage of alternative medicine. Though life has thrown me many curveballs, and at times I felt like giving up, there are many people to whom I will forever be indebted for my success. This book is dedicated to all of you.

Contents

Acknowledgments

I especially wish to thank my patients of the last thirty-four years who have encouraged me to investigate and learn alternative health care. Through their suggestions, advice and positive response, I have been encouraged to continue alternative therapies in spite of peer pressure and criticism. At their persuasion, I was also encouraged to write this book, and several of them have unselfishly helped in typing, critiquing and editing the text.

I am grateful to Dr. R. G. Williams for being my first employer and instructing me in surgery. Equally valuable, he taught me the importance of a good bedside manner.

For their loyalty and love, I want to give my heartfelt thanks to Bob and Alice Artibee, Dianne Chaperon, Harry Eidenier, Carole Anne Franklin, Kaye Porter, David and Gail Reeves, Steve Steiner and Darwin Teos. They reviewed, suggested revisions and spent considerable time critiquing this book. To Jan Boylan my greatest thanks for typing and retyping many times to get the book in its final form, to Bob Artibee who suggested the book's title and to Carolyn Baker for the artwork on the book's cover. With people like these in their lives, all physicians would be as fortunate as I am.

Foreword

When my old and dear friend Dr. Gene Schroeder asked me to write the foreward for this book, I was both delighted and honored to be asked by one of the most talented, caring and honest healers I have had the pleasure of knowing in my thirty years of work in the healing arts.

Although opinions may differ on the what, why and how of this book, in my opinion, it is the story of one doctor's journey from traditional medicine to patient-oriented holistic medicine and what he found most useful for his patients along the way.

As Dr. Schroeder indicates in the text, only brief descriptions are given for the various therapies, modalities, supplements and so forth listed in the book. The purpose of this book is to introduce the reader to the things he found to have value (many of which he taught to me), with the hope that the reader will go on to further investigate these therapies in their pursuit of improved health.

This book provides us with a guide, written in clear and understandable language, that gives us clear direction in how to avoid and overcome bad food, bad water, bad medicine and so on. Because we continue to place more and more chemicals into our water, air, soil, foods and, therefore, our bodies, this book is needed now more than ever.

This book is a must read for anyone who wants to know more about how to help themselves stay healthy or return to a state of true health.

Harry O. Eidenier, Jr., Ph.D.

Preface

Since the late sixties I have been called a quack because I dared to dream and treat patients with other methods, remedies and programs that were not advised or accepted by traditional, conventional medicine. Several ideas I advocated then, which I do not fully discuss in this book, are widely accepted now, thirty years later—early ambulation of surgical patients, the use of physician assistants, high-fiber diets and the use of magnesium therapy. Being ahead of the crowd is always risky, an opportunity for advanced thinkers to be called quacks. The term quack has been used by those physicians who have not taken the time or energy to become familiar with alternative therapy. They portray all alternative physicians as snake oil salesmen. The only quack I am familiar with is the person who knowingly promotes an unwise remedy or treatment program strictly for its financial benefit.

I believe you need to learn about the many alternative therapies so that you may avail yourself of them when the need arises. Through this book I hope to acquaint you with several alternative choices to treat or maintain your health. I believe in fostering wellness rather than treating illness. Each person is unique and must be evaluated and treated as such. There are many different methods of treatment in addition to allopathic medicine, the traditional, medically accepted approach. Allopathic therapies do not adequately treat a number of illnesses, both chronic and acute. Consequently, I began using alternative methods more than thirty years ago and because I have been successful using integrated therapies, I continue to investigate further possibilities. By using alternative methods of treatment I have been able to lower my hospital medical admission rate from more than three hundred a year to less than three a year.

When I first entered this type of practice, it was called "alternative," meaning a choice other than an allopathic practice (conventional, such as medical or osteopathic). Other names have since been attributed to alternative therapies. *Preventive medicine* describes a doctor and patient focusing on ways an individual can improve his attitudes, exercise, breathing, nutrition, lifestyle and, therefore, the results of physical examinations. Such an approach will ensure the best opportunity of living a long, healthy life.

Holistic medicine includes the treatment of the entire person by evaluating the patient's history, physical exam and laboratory tests as well as social, emotional, sexual, spiritual and family factors. Oftentimes specific counseling can be more beneficial than a prescription. Holistic medicine is a term that can and should be used for both allopathic and alternative medicine. Unfortunately, it is rarely used in most allopathic offices today.

Complementary medicine is another term used to describe an alternative approach to medicine. It accurately pictures the desire and intention of alternative physicians to augment treatment methods accepted in allopathic medicine and not to replace them. It is the best way to depict what I have been trying to do in my humble way to bridge the gap between traditional and alternative medicine. The most recent term, *Integrated medicine*, encompasses this philosophy.

The purpose of this book is to familiarize you with different methods of preventing and treating illness. I believe we need both allopathic and alternative methods of treatment. I want to do my part to bring these two philosophies of medicine together. At the time I began practicing alternative medicine, the two philosophies were worlds apart. Because of tremendous economic pressures, organized allopathic medicine is starting to listen and learn.

According to a new study from Beth Israel Deaconess Medical Center in Boston, eighty-three million Americans spent twenty-seven billion dollars on alternative therapies in 1997. To protect their market share, the big drug companies are starting to enter the alternative market by promoting and selling herbal and homeopathic products. The American Medical Association has even embraced the idea of alternative therapies by devoting their entire November 11, 1998, publication, the *Journal of the American Medical Association,* to exploring alternative therapies. Over fifty percent of medical schools now offer courses in alternative therapies.

I predict this open-minded thinking will promote more study and research. I am grateful to the Boy Scouts of America for the motto To Make the Best Better, which has encouraged me to look for better ways to do things with an open mind. Medical practitioners must realize we are individuals and treat us accordingly. What works for one person may not work for another. Unfortunately, most research is based on the effectiveness of a given therapy on groups of patients rather than on individuals.

This book will help you to more fully appreciate the role alternative therapies can play in your health and longevity. I have purposely limited my discussion of the various alternative therapies so as not to overwhelm you but rather to stimulate your interest. I hope you will be interested enough to pursue a topic and learn more about it. There are many audiotapes, videos and books available on all the subjects discussed. Think happy thoughts, be positive and be willing to change for your overall betterment. Read with an open mind and let your intuition be your guide.

My peers in the medical world have often labeled me a witch doctor, a rebel and even a quack. I may be a rebel, but I am not a quack, and the proof can be found in my story. I hope you benefit from it.

Chapter 1

My Journey of Spirit

I was born November 30, 1934, under the sun sign of Sagittarius in Bay City, Michigan, with my moon in Virgo and Venus also in Sagittarius. I was the first child of wonderful parents, Esther and Walter Carl Schroeder. My mother, a farm girl, had waited until her late twenties to marry. My father was a barber, and also had other occupations during the Depression, such as foreman of the Works Progress Administration (WPA). When I was about a year old, I had to start wearing glasses because of strabismus, that is, crossed eyes, and because of my young age, my glasses had to be held on with a black elastic band. Maybe that was the reason I would see things differently throughout my lifetime. As a youngster, I was perhaps not any different from any other boy of my age. However, I did have, as I stated, very caring parents who also believed in discipline. My father did not hesitate to use a leather shaving belt when it was needed. I was a child who valued independence and possessed a personal belief system, both of which caused me to have undue problems for my age. But for the most part all of my childhood memories are happy.

On my first day of kindergarten I remember going off behind the old red brick Lincoln School in Bay City, Michigan, and swearing under the fire escape to show that now I was grown up and I could be more on my own and do what I wanted. My brother Gary was two years younger, and then following him by two years, came my sister Janice.

We lived in Brooks, a suburb of Bay City, and it was there that I got my first dog, a cocker spaniel. When I asked my mother whether the dog was a boy or girl, she told me it was a boy. So I named him Boy. He became a devoted companion to me for the next fourteen years. Not only did Boy bring me my bedroom slippers on command but he also turned out to be an excellent pheasant-hunting dog when I was older. Another memory from living in Brooks was of my brother and me: although barely old enough to pull a little red wagon, we would travel around the neighborhood selling strawberries.

We moved from Brooks to Columbus Avenue in Bay City, where my father built a home. We arrived there in time for me to start kindergarten and also to hear the announcement on the radio that World War II had begun.

In the summer after my first grade we moved to a small farm of sixty acres in Lincoln, Michigan, about one hundred miles north of Bay City. My father was working as a barber inspector for the state of Michigan. At school they gave me a test and decided I could skip the second grade and so, without difficulty, I promptly went into the third grade. (In the fourth, fifth and sixth grades I learned how to play chess but, alas, I haven't played it since.)

Because of my glasses, I was often ridiculed and called Four-eyes. As a consequence, I became somewhat introverted, but I continued to do well in school. Sometimes I would be beaten up by my schoolmates and, occasionally, by my older cousins. I remember one incident where I was angry enough to actually beat up a bully who was killing a nest of garter snakes. I just couldn't understand why someone would be killing something that was harmless and defenseless.

My father, an excellent hunter and fisherman, taught us hunting and fishing skills that we eagerly put into practice. My mother, although totally against killing anything, took my brother and me fishing many times. Our first fishing ventures were for rock bass, blue gills and largemouth bass, which we caught by wading out into nearby Brownlee Lake. One day while fishing for rock bass with a homemade six-foot pole with the line wrapped on two nails, I snagged a big largemouth bass on its side and, unbelievably, landed it. From then on, I have been a died-in-the wool, forever-and-ever fisherman. About one-third of our farm was in swamp and woodland, and it was a wonderful haven for partridge, that is, ruffed grouse, and snowshoe rabbits and a sprinkling of cottontails.

One snowy day when my brother and I were in our swamp hunting rabbits, he shot his first one. I think he was only about seven at the time. He proudly marched into the kitchen and showed my mother his first rabbit. She scolded him saying, "How could you have the heart to kill a poor little rabbit?" He thought for a while and then he answered, "But, momma, this was a bad, bad rabbit."

Thus began our many days and years of hunting and fishing experiences that we still talk about from time to time. I quit hunting four years ago, however, and probably will only hunt again if I find myself in need of food.

After completing the eighth grade at Lincoln, I had to transfer to Oscoda High School, which was a twenty-mile bus ride every morning. I continued to be somewhat reserved throughout high school even though I was well liked. I did well in my studies and graduated as valedictorian, much to the surprise of the teachers and my school companions. In high school I began having my first and probably mild psychic experiences even though I did not recognize them as such for a long time. The first psychic intuitive experience I finally recognized was when my friend Walter Buzek had an accident with his car. He had gone over a hill off the road and some months later as I was driving by the same spot I thought to myself, "I think I'll stop and see where Walter went off the road." I stopped my car, got out and walked over to the steep hill and found at the bottom where the crash had ended. I didn't think anything about it at the time other than having explored the spot where he had ruined his vehicle, which I believe was a 1934 Plymouth. Sometime later I thought about it and wondered how I knew to stop the car and look at that particular spot. No one had ever told me where the accident had happened, and there were no signs on the road indicating there had been one. He had just gone off the road and over a hill. I probably had had other psychic encounters prior to this, but this was the first that I can remember.

After high school I attended a junior college in Bay City, Michigan, and at that time my personality did a flip-flop. From being an introvert, I suddenly became an extrovert. My goal in life was to be a research chemist, so I took the courses that were necessary to lead up to that degree. My mother had wanted me to be a medical doctor. I don't ever recall her telling me why. There had never been one in the family, but it was her dream and always her goal for me. As she persisted in her dream, the dream began to take a hold of me. So I also registered in some premedical classes, and after two years of junior college, in 1954, I entered the University of Michigan, where I spent two more years working not only on chemistry but also on my premedical requirements. To be on the safe side, I also took courses in education, thinking that maybe someday I could become a chemistry teacher.

Between my junior and senior years at Michigan, I married Shirlee May Arndt, from Bay City. She was going to school at Northeastern College in Ypsilanti, Michigan. For a semester we lived in the married couples housing area at Ann Arbor, and it was there that one night I had an experience I remember quite vividly to this day. As we were lying in bed, I said to Shirlee, "I'll certainly be glad when you give me that watch you bought for me." She looked startled and then she quickly denied that she was giving me a watch, but I closed my eyes and could see the watch in great detail. I told her the name of the watch, its color, shape, and the fact that it had a leather band. I gave her all of the characteristics of the watch, but she still denied that she had bought me one. The next night as we were again lying in bed, I thought of the watch, and told her I would be glad when she gave it to me. Again, she denied buying it. I went on to tell her where and when she had bought the watch, the name of the store, the city and then I finally told her the price she had paid for it. Apparently, this was too much because she jumped out of bed, ran into the next room, got the watch and sales slip and returned to bed to show it to me. It was just as I had seen it in my mind's eye. However, I was a little bit wrong: the price of the watch was off by one penny.

From that moment on, I was convinced there was more to our senses than the conventional ones to which we ascribed. I knew there was something more there. I didn't know what it was; people didn't talk about it, but I knew there was something more.

I applied for medical school after my junior year at the University of Michigan. I interviewed with Dr. Whitaker, the assistant dean, but I was turned down. I finished my senior year and received my bachelor degree in chemistry. I reapplied for medical school and again was interviewed by Dr. Whitaker. He started to ask me questions, but I replied that he had asked me the same questions the year before, so I suggested he should ask me something different. Understandably, he became somewhat agitated and told me my grades were borderline. I would not learn whether I would be accepted for three months, when the next semester grades were available. I became upset. I told him that I wanted to get into medical school and that I would get in regardless of his opinions. One thing led to another and he finally got so angry he ordered me out of his office. Another potential student was in the waiting room and he had heard some of the dialogue. He was scared and asked me whether he dared go in there. He did and was accepted and ended up being my lab partner. And, by the way, one week later, not three months, much to my surprise and elation, I received notification of my acceptance to medical school. Needless to say, I was very happy.

In medical school many of my instructors did not know my regular name—they only knew me as Slash. (Perhaps the fastest knife in anatomy class.)

Was that a sign of things to come? Who knows? I studied all the right things and managed to pass the tests.

After my first year of medical school, my lab partner asked me to join him in taking the state licensing exam. I was surprised that he wanted to do this because the exam covered all four years of medical school and we had just finished our first year! He persuaded me to try because we would be taking the test soon after completing anatomy and several other difficult courses, and it would be easier to take the exam then, rather than waiting three more years. After all, he reasoned, the tests that we failed could be retaken at the regular time. From our class of nearly two hundred we were the only two to attempt this feat. We were truly amazed when we got our test results. He had passed every test! I had passed every test except pathology. My grade was a sixty-eight and I needed a seventy to pass. In my sophomore year I had pathology for the entire year. When I took the exam after my fourth year, I only passed it with a seventy-eight.

In medical school I felt somewhat different from my fellow classmates. I felt there was something more to healing people than giving them medications. I often questioned why we studied some of these rare illnesses we might never see again. And, why didn't we spend more time learning about the belief systems of patients?

I learned about the placebo effect in an orthopedic ward on from a patient who couldn't sleep and was distraught because he was hung up on ropes, harnesses and weights. I convinced him that a placebo pill would help him sleep very soundly and much to my amazement it worked beautifully.

I wondered why we didn't get instructions on nutrition because, after all, the way we eat is so important. The way we exercise is just as important. And certainly the way we breathe is important. Why were we not offered classes in these basic fundamentals?

I saw failures in our treatment programs even at a time when I considered the University of Michigan to be one of the finest teaching and healing institutions in the world. I saw failures and I wondered why; why did we have failures?

The failure I remember most vividly was a patient by the name of Mrs. Connolly. I became acquainted with her when I was on the private service of one of the leading medical professors at the University of Michigan. I was very fortunate to be chosen as one of the medical students to spend a month on his rotation. Mrs. Connolly was there an entire month being evaluated for chronic diarrhea. We became good friends. She was a country/western singer. Her husband worked as a repairman for Shakespeare fishing equipment and since I was an avid fisherman, I had plenty of fishing reels that needed repair. So he repaired them, and he even gave me new reels, lines and other equipment but I was upset when she left the hospital after a month of evaluations but with no answers for her problem. We'll talk about her later when we discuss food allergies.

Before graduating from the University of Michigan, I had to take an externship and I chose St. Luke's Hospital in Saginaw, Michigan. While there I made good friends with the pathologist and became even more interested in doing research. I had spent the previous two summers at the University of Michigan doing research in the Pediatrics Laboratory under the guidance and counseling of

Dr. Tsao. My experiments were related to enzyme electrophoresis, and even though I made a number of new discoveries, for some reason I did not publish my results.

While at St. Luke's Hospital I became intrigued in the use of hypnosis. One of the doctors in the emergency room was quite proficient at it and he showed me the many ways it could be used in a regular practice as well as in emergency situations. The first time I saw it actually put to good use was when a young girl came in with a severely lacerated tongue. The doctor proceeded to hypnotize her and then asked her to stick out her tongue. She held it out while he very deftly sutured the very serious laceration without any disturbance from the girl. She experienced no pain during the procedure. I was hooked—I definitely wanted to learn hypnosis. This was my first introduction to alternative medicine, since hypnosis was not really regarded as a tool for medicine at that time. This was 1959.

My medical practice journey finally began in June of 1960 on a warm and beautiful day in Ann Arbor, Michigan, when I graduated from the University of Michigan Medical School. Little did I realize how my thoughts about medicine would change in the years to come. When I look back, I realize there were a number of factors that helped me to embrace holistic (alternative, preventative, complementary, integrative) medicine.

The fact that I grew up on a farm enabled me to appreciate the nutritional aspects of medicine. I knew we had to use the right types of soil and fertilizers to nourish plants so they would grow properly. Our animals needed the proper balance in their feed. If they were fed inferior products, we knew they would not be healthy. When we fed our animals and crops properly, there was very little disease. The mineral content of the soil is essential to crop, animal and, subsequently, human health. This relationship is not fully appreciated. As early as the midthirties the U.S. Department of Agriculture pronounced our soils deficient in minerals. If our soils are deficient, our food will also be deficient. Since medical school, I have found that mineral deficiencies play a large role in illness. The only way we can ensure the proper amounts is through supplementation.

Most doctors are well aware of the benefits of sodium and potassium, but have only recently considered the value of magnesium, a common mineral. I have been trying to get my colleagues to use magnesium for toxemia of childbirth, premature labor, cardiac arrhythmia, constipation, muscle cramping and more. It has only been in recent years that the general medical community has accepted its benefits. It literally took me several years before I was able to persuade our hospital laboratory to include magnesium in a routine analysis along with sodium and potassium. In order to correctly identify magnesium deficiency, red blood cell magnesium must be analyzed. (Selenium is another important mineral found to be an important factor in prevention of cancer, aneurysms and heart disease.)

My farm experience has had a positive effect on my acceptance of nutrition as a form of therapy. My father's use of chiropractic and his belief in it encouraged me to investigate chiropractic as a means of therapy. I also give my mother credit for advising me to always keep an open mind and to try things before forming an opinion. That attitude has engendered my belief that the art of medicine is just as important as the science of medicine.

After graduation I went to Borgess Hospital in Kalamazoo, Michigan, in an excellent rotating internship, a one-year program. When I finished the internship I was fully prepared to enter the general practice of medicine without feeling the need to go on for further study. The attending staff at the hospital were wonderful; interns did not have to do a lot of basic unnecessary work and they were quick to call us in on important cases. We didn't even have to do histories and physicals, which were a real pain for interns. We were able to spend our time actually doing the more active evaluation and treatment. In addition to seeing patients at the hospital we were able to go to individual practices to work. On one occasion I was able to take over a doctor's office for a week and see his patients while he was gone. This was an almost unheard of practice at the time. I also was able to deliver more than 450 babies and so my interest was definitely kindled for obstetrics, and I found it a very rewarding part of the practice. I had wanted to be a surgeon since I'd decided to go to medical school. The surgeons at the University of Michigan, however, were usually disenchanted with what they called LMDs, or local physicians, and their ability to practice medicine. Because of this I made a vow to myself that instead of becoming a surgeon I would be one of those LMDs and demonstrate that I could be a good medical doctor.

During my internship I was called by the United States Army to go to Detroit to have a physical to see if I was qualified for service. I had been very sick twice with infectious hepatitis during junior college. The army arranged for a Greyhound bus to take a group of us from Kalamazoo to Detroit, and it was on that Greyhound ride that another aspect of my psychic ability proved itself. I had long wondered about mental telepathy and pondered whether such a thing existed. On the way to Detroit I put it to the test to find out if it worked. You will read the answer in the chapter on psychic ability (intuition).

It was during my year of internship that I read a book on hypnosis. It was written in such a way that it scared me away from using it clinically, for the time being.

During that year I was privileged to have as one of my attending physicians, Dr. James Breneman, who was excellent at diagnosing and treating food allergies. His teachings drove home the point about the importance of diagnosing food allergies at a time when such allergies were not well recognized.

Following my internship, in 1961, I moved to the Upper Peninsula of Michigan to a small mining town named Ishpeming. I went into practice with R. G. Williams, M.D., a general practitioner and an excellent surgeon. Our association lasted until his death. Before he died we had several other physicians join our clinic, including Dr. Lou Rosenbaum, a general practitioner, and Dr. Martin Lexmond, a general surgeon. Under their supervision I was given daily instruction in surgery and was eventually able to do some general surgery on my own. Dr. Swamy, a cardiologist, also joined our group several years later. I considered him one of my best friends, but I was never able to convince him of the value of nutritional therapies. He was a true allopathic physician and resisted trying alternative methods. I failed in trying to convince him of the benefits even though I continued the effort right up until his death.

I give credit to Dr. Williams for teaching me bedside manner, one of the most important arts of medical practice—sometimes more so than its science.

In 1966 at thirty-two years of age I was drafted out of private practice and into the United States Air Force. After basic training in Wichita Falls, at Shepard Air Force Base, I was sent to Grand Forks Air Base in Grand Forks, North Dakota. At first I was somewhat unhappy because I'd asked to be placed at either an air base in eastern upper Michigan or in Alaska. Both of my requests obviously had been turned down. By that time I had been in private practice for five years, and had more practical experience than any other medical officer on the base with the exception of the commander. I enjoyed working at the base and especially one aspect of it: I did not have to worry about people being able to afford their prescriptions because whatever we prescribed the Air Force would furnish. There were some limitations. I worked as a general medical officer and worked some nights in the emergency room. I also rotated through the obstetrical department. When I broke a hand playing softball, I was eliminated from obstetrical practice, which was fine with me because delivering babies didn't quite fit into my schedule.

One day as I was browsing through the library I ran across a small book on hypnosis written by an anesthesiologist. It quickened my interest in hypnosis again, and I decided to try it. I figured out a few relaxation techniques, and lo and behold, I found it was quite easy to do. I started treating patients and got amazing results. This was after the widely publicized story in the fifties and sixties of a person, known as Bridey Murphy, being regressed under hypnosis. I thought that since someone else had been able to do it, I could try as well, so I regressed patients into former lifetimes and became very successful with it. I hypnotized many other people with various problems with excellent results, and I will relate several of their stories in the chapter on hypnosis.

During my two years at Grand Forks, I noticed a dramatic increase in my intuitive abilities. Why they occurred then I do not know. Perhaps it was because I was doing a lot of hypnosis; perhaps it was the area, perhaps it was because of my noon hour meditations. I did not know the reason then and I still do not know. However, I had many psychic (intuitive) experiences that further proved to me that the brain has many functions of which we are not usually aware.

In the spring of 1968 my marriage ended in an amicable divorce. I left the air force in the fall of 1968. I returned to private practice in Ishpeming, Michigan, at the end of 1968, still associated with Dr. Lou Rosenbaum, Dr. Martin Lexmond and Dr. Reginald Williams. I continued to practice obstetrics, pediatrics, general medicine and surgery.

After being single for two years, I married a former patient I had met in Grand Forks. Her name was Barbara. I met her at the emergency room at the air force base. When she came in she was a *status asthmaticus*. With all our available drugs, we were not able to stop her asthmatic attack, so I resorted to hypnosis and amazingly it stopped the attack immediately. She was very much impressed, as were the emergency room personnel and I. The next time I saw her she was again in the emergency room in an asthmatic episode. We again used hypnosis and subsequently gave her other hypnosis treatments. To my knowledge she is still without significant asthmatic difficulties except for some mild symptoms with exertion.

After a year back from the air force, I met a person named Charley Dodge, from whom I learned a great deal about nutritional supplementation. He told me how people could be treated using nutritional products, namely products from Standard Process Laboratories. I was very skeptical, so we did some experiments on volunteers, giving them various nutritional supplements—with dramatic improvement.

At that point in time, at the end of 1969, I started treating various conditions with nutritional supplements and much to my amazement, I noticed good results, especially with conditions that were not amenable to traditional therapy. About the same time I attended a workshop in kinesiology directed by Dr. Bruce West. At the beginning, I was totally skeptical. However, as the seminar went on I was amazed at the responses from many people. Until then I had looked upon it more as a gimmick, though an interesting phenomenon. Afterward I would demonstrate it for various people but would never include it in any therapy or treatment program, or even use it as a diagnostic tool. Over the next twenty years I would periodically be reminded of kinesiology, but I never attempted to study it in detail. It was not until around 1990 that I started using kinesiology for diagnosis and treatment. We'll talk more about it in a later chapter.

For approximately the next eighteen years, from 1969 to 1987, I continued to work at the Williams Clinic at Ishpeming. As the years passed, I became more and more proficient at nutritional therapy, and explored the use of various nutritional supplements for different conditions. I continued to be amazed by the results.

During this period I also used hypnosis with good results—on an individual basis and in group sessions. Probably because of the many psychic experiences I had had at Grand Forks Air Force Base, I started collecting a large library of psychic literature. In particular I enjoyed thoroughly the various books written about Edgar Cayce and his abilities. (Without telling anyone, I wished that someday I could do some of the things he has accomplished.) Not only did Cayce have tremendous psychic abilities, but he also devised different alternative therapies that could be used for many medical conditions.

I continued to have many psychic experiences, and one that stands out in my mind was an incident that happened while I was playing softball in Michigan. I was playing center field and lost a very expensive sapphire ring. I stopped the game and had both teams come out onto the field to help me find it. But we failed.

Sometime later I got the idea of trying to teleport my ring because I had read that it was possible in certain cases. So I began focusing my thoughts on the ring's return. Within two weeks after starting the meditation, I walked into my son's bedroom, opened up his closet door (where I had some hunting equipment) and couldn't believe my eyes: there was the ring on a shelf!

As the years progressed from 1969 to 1987, I continued my general practice using progressively more and more nutritional therapy and less and less hypnosis, although I continued using hypnosis for childbirth, phobias, asthma and numerous other medical conditions.

On one occasion I used it in a legal case that I thought was somewhat unusual. A young man had killed a storekeeper in the process of a robbery and the authorities were trying to determine whether it was a first-degree or second-degree murder. We regressed him under hypnosis and recorded his story. We also questioned him under sodium pentothal and found that the two stories corroborated. We then were able to use these stories in court in his defense, and because of the regression and sodium pentothal analysis, he received a second-degree murder conviction rather than first-degree. I was quite surprised that the court allowed this testimony, but nevertheless it did happen.

During this period of time I also became aware of two other types of alternative medicine. The first was foot reflexology, which was an additional technique I used to help in the diagnosis of various problems. The second was intravenous and oral chelation, which I learned after much prompting from Dave Bennett, a very close friend who had developed coronary artery disease and subsequently had a coronary bypass. This opened the door for me to a totally new concept of treating heart disease, and it has proven very useful to my patients ever since.

I was also very active in the winter sport of snowmobiling during this period and joined a cross-country snowmobile club. The club was called the Peninsula Pathfinders, and we rode many hundreds of miles on snowmobiles. We traveled from the Upper Peninsula of Michigan all the way to West Yellowstone on snowmobiles. Another year we went from the Upper Peninsula to Portland, Maine, by the same method, and yet another year we did a gypsy ride and went to Hudson Bay on snowmobiles. These were our three longest trips, although we had many shorter trips interspersed.

I had originally injured my right knee practicing judo in the air force and thereafter had recurrent problems with the knee whenever I played volleyball. Finally, I started having back pains that were so severe at times that I had to crawl on my hands and knees to go the bathroom or get up and down stairs. I was on crutches a good deal of the time. Though it was difficult, I continued to assist and do general surgery and even deliver babies while on my crutches.

In the 1970s I met a gentleman by the name of Roy Massner, who was also very much interested in alternative medicine. We subsequently developed an organization called the SURE Institute, whose purpose was to encourage the formation of alternative medicine clinics throughout the United States. We had our professional office in Dallas and held meetings there with practitioners of different fields of alternative medicine. On one of these occasions, we held a seminar and I traveled to Dallas on my crutches. When I got there late in the afternoon, I met with Roy and he introduced me to his brother Ray, who was a chiropractor in Prescott, Arizona. When he saw that I was in distress, he asked me to let his brother do some chiropractic on my back. I said that I really didn't believe in chiropractors, even though my father had gone to them all his life. With this in the back of my mind, I was persuaded to let Ray Massner adjust me. I will tell you more about it in the chapter on chiropractors.

This was my introduction to the fourth form of alternative medicine, chiropractic. (The first was hypnosis, the second nutrition and the third, foot reflexology.) The fifth was chelation therapy, which I learned at the urging of a close friend. Subsequently, I started referring patients with back problems to chiropractors with good results. I saw a very great many back injuries because much of our clinic's work was emergency service for the Cleveland Cliffs Iron Company, which at that time had about five thousand employees whoworked in the company's iron mines in Ishpeming.

I felt very lonesome in the Upper Peninsula doing alternative medicine because I was the only physician within three hundred miles doing this type of practice, integrating it with my general practice. I was called everything from a quack to a crazy doctor. My patients, however, continued to feel otherwise.

I had remarried for the third time. My first two marriages had each lasted thirteen years, and I was determined this one would last. My third wife, Kathleen, was the daughter of a surgical nurse, one with whom I had worked for twenty-five years at Bell Memorial Hospital in Ishpeming. She has two sons, Adam and Andy. I consider myself to be very fortunate to have married such a wonderful person and still be in good relationships with my two previous wives. I believe this is very important because we have children together. Elizabeth, Laurie and Jeffrey were with Shirlee, my first wife, and Stephen was with Barbara, my second wife. I also adopted Barbara's daughter Katherine.

With my third beautiful wife I have now broken the thirteen-year jinx and have been married for eighteen years, with no end in sight. I have learned a great deal from my previous marriages and divorces. I believe I have learned to communicate better, be more understanding, considerate and forgiving. I hope I have gained some wisdom. I believe my experiences have given me insight so that I can be a better husband and a better counselor to my patients. I strongly believe that one of the major problems in the world today is poor communication; it is something we all need to work on to improve our lives.

During my last ten years in Ishpeming, before I moved to Arizona, I was getting more and more fed up with the medical environment, the American Medical Association and their position against alternative medicine, the changes in the insurance companies, and the restrictions on patient hospital stays. All in all, medicine was just not what it had been in the sixties and early seventies. Many of my fellow physicians in the Marquette, Michigan, area also felt the way I did in that medicine no longer gave them the enjoyment it had previously. I was a member of many state and national physician-review committees, and I spent a great deal of my extra time sitting on a variety of other boards and committees. All in all, I was unhappy with the direction in which I perceived medicine was heading. Therefore, in 1987, after the Supreme Court *Wilkes* decision, an antitrust suit that made it possible for M.D.s to associate with chiropractors, I elected to move my practice to Prescott, Arizona. I entered a combined practice with Dr. Ray Massner, who had been giving my back such excellent care for the previous ten years. In Prescott I had decided not to work in the hospital or practice any further surgery or obstetrics, but to just do general practice, office based only. This would rid myself of all the hospital requirements like attendance at meetings and so forth.

As I was starting my practice, one of the Prescott internists suggested that to aid my practice growth, I might consider doing work for the Arizona Health Care Cost Containment System (AHCCCS), which was a type of Medicaid for the state of Arizona. I readily accepted, and worked for AHCCCS for one year until AHCCCS discovered I was not on a hospital staff. They had been doing regular reviews on all of my cases and were impressed. They always gave me a 100 percent review. They asked me if I would apply for privileges at the local hospital so that I could continue to work for AHCCCS. Although not wanting privileges, I applied to the hospital as a means of gaining additional time to treat AHCCCS patients.

I had informed various members of the medical staff at the hospital that when I was accepted, I would refuse the privileges because I did not want to become a hospital staff member. They gave me an oral examination with about fifteen doctors present. Later they gave me a written examination that they claimed I failed. I disagreed, asked for a hearing, and they reluctantly agreed. At the hearing one of the local doctors admitted under oath that the reason I was rejected was because I was working with a chiropractor. Also under oath, another doctor refused to inform me what questions I had answered incorrectly. To sum up, rather than fight them, inasmuch as I did not want the privileges of the hospital anyway, I agreed to withdraw my application.

They had suggested that unless I did so, they would report my failure to obtain a hospital license to the state board. I had to give up my AHCCCS patients, but as it turned out, it was a good move anyway because AHCCCS had refused to pay me for a number of cases. That was what other doctors had also experienced. When I subsequently left AHCCCS, they still owed me several thousand dollars. I do not expect to be paid.

Dr. Massner, in addition to doing his chiropractic work, also practiced homeopathy and acupuncture. I was quite impressed with his results and when I discovered that there was a homeopathic medical society in Arizona, I began attending their meetings. This was wonderful because I was able to associate with other doctors who believed and practiced alternative medicine: I finally felt I was not alone. I studied homeopathy, took my licensure exam and received my homeopathic license in April of 1993. I could now practice alternative medicine in Arizona, which at that time was only one of three states in the United States to have a board of homeopathic medicine.

So homeopathy was a sixth addition to my alternative practice. I realized that many doctors felt this was a placebo type medicine because the theory behind homeopathic medicine was totally opposite allopathic medicine. Homeopathy was somewhat difficult for me to understand and accept inasmuch as I had earned a bachelor of science degree in chemistry from Ann Arbor prior to entering medical school. It was not long before I was convinced that homeopathic medicine was not a placebo but had a very valuable place as one of the alternatives to allopathic medicine. Homeopathic medicine is based on the Laws of Similars. A couple of cases I had early in my homeopathic practice persuaded me that homeopathic medicine did work and could not be explained by anything else for its success.

Having a number of these alternative therapies available makes me feel like a carpenter who has more than two tools in his tool case. I believe patients need to be treated the way they want to be treated. They respond better, are more responsible with their medication schedule and get much better overall results.

I next studied Reiki and took the various attunements over approximately a two-year span. Reiki is similar to "laying on of hands" with the exception that it has sacred symbols that are also used. Reiki can be done near and far, similar to evaluating by kinesiology. I do not do much Reiki because of the time involved. However, my goal is to do instantaneous Reiki to get immediate results. I've had at least two episodes where by just touching the patients, I've corrected their symptoms. This is not Reiki per se. In one case a tall fellow who couldn't swallow even his own saliva had been in the emergency room all night. I had not seen him before, but just by standing behind him and touching his throat was able to helo him swallow immediately, much to the amazement of both of us. The second case was a friend who was visiting and had just stopped by the office to say good-bye. She was having severe back pain at the time. Unaware of the pain, I laid my hand on her back and it wasn't until she was down the road a block or two that she realized the pain was gone.

I also took courses in bio-oxidative medicine and have used intravenous hydrogen peroxide with good results in acute infections and emphysema. I now have restarted chelation after a long hiatus. After I came to Arizona I asked the medical board if I could do chelation therapy and they said no. So for a number of years I did not give it here as I had in Michigan. I was able to restart chelation therapy after obtaining my homeopathic medical license.

The Arizona Board of Medicine, that is, Bomex, evaluated my patient records for pain prescriptions and they thought I was giving out too much pain medicine. They reprimanded me and made me take a course in pain management. They later reviewed my records again. They found I was using B_{12} for other than pernicious anemia, and that I was using colchicine for back cases, which they did not approve of in spite of medical literature attesting to its value. They also found I was using an herbal brown salve that clears ninety-nine percent of skin cancer in one or two applications.

They put a restriction on my license directing me not to use any colchicine, B_{12} or brown salve. The only condition for which I could use B_{12} was pernicious anemia, which is somewhat ridiculous. I have since petitioned the board with a considerable number of medical articles regarding the use of B_{12} for other than pernicious anemia, and finally I have been allowed to use it. In the fall of 1997, I petitioned the board to allow me to use chelation, and they referred me to the homeopathic board that heartily endorsed its use. This was very good because it is beneficial for many vascular problems, in heavy metal detoxification and for antiaging. Bomex, in an effort to rid the state of an alternative doctor, asked me to take a special (spex) exam and stated that if I failed it, they would take my license away. However, even if they had, I still would have been able to practice under my homeopathic license. To make a long story short, I passed the exam, much to their surprise, and since that time I have had no further confrontations with the Bomex Board.

In July of 1997 I accepted the position of physician for the Gerson Clinic near Sedona, Arizona. I had been familiar with the Gerson therapy for at least seventeen years, since I had first met Charlotte Gerson at a meeting of our SURE organization in Dallas. She was carrying on the work of her father, Max Gerson. This is an alternative type of therapy using detoxification with organic food and organic juices in addition to coffee and chamomile enemas. The therapy also consists of using potassium, hydrochloric acid, pancreatease, thyroid extracts, iodine and various other herbals and mineral supplements. It is a very effective detoxification program and good not only for cancer but also for many other major diseases that improve with detoxification. I worked there one day a week for a year.

I am now in solo practiceat the Rainbow Wellness Clinic, 843 Miller Valley Road, Prescott, Arizona 86301—Phone (928) 717-0678; Fax (928) 717-0712. I am not affiliated with any hospital. In the rare case where a patient needs to be hospitalized, I refer him or her to an appropriate specialist. I do general practice and minor surgery in the office. I specialize in holistic medicine for all ages. A number of the alternative therapies that I find very beneficial are discussed later.

Since I first started practicing holistic medicine, there has been a great shift toward its acceptance by the American public and, more slowly, by traditional physicians. It is very gratifying to see this change in consciousness.

Since 1970 I have wanted to establish a holistic/alternative clinic but have financially been unable to do so. In the early 1990s we established a holistic medical corporation called The Rainbow Medicine Lodge. Plans for a unique building were drawn with an Indian motif. Operational plans were established. The concept is to have traditional physicians of different specialties work in association with holistic physicians who use various alternative methods. Patients would be assured of the best of all therapies for their individual case. A board of all physicians would review difficult cases. It is envisioned that the Rainbow Medicine Lodge would also be used as a teaching center not only for physicians but also for auxiliary medical personnel. Unfortunately, we have not been able to obtain the necessary funding to realize our dream, but we believe it will become available when the time is right. We would be more than grateful for any financial gifts to our Rainbow Medicine Lodge Corporation that would hasten the day our goal of a holistic integrated medical clinic could be a reality.

Another part of our concept is to be able to treat Native Americans at our clinic. The president of our corporation, Carole Franklin, is one-half Sauk and Fox. Her father was a medicine man in Oklahoma, and she was forced to attend a government Indian school there. We feel that most Native Americans would be more comfortable being treated with alternative therapies. We also plan on having a medicine man on the staff of our clinic when it is operational.

Chapter 2

The Art of Medicine

The art of medicine is the manner in which a good doctor treats his patients. Doctors must have the ability to be good listeners. This skill is essential to making a diagnosis. The patient must be allowed to discuss his symptoms. This is a form of treatment in itself. When the patient can talk to his doctor without feeling intimidated or threatened, he will be more likely to comply with their suggestions.

The doctor should not only be a good listener, but also kind, patient and at times humorous. He or she must be willing to answer the patient's questions and not be judgmental. The doctor should be open-minded and unbiased.

Physicians should treat the patient and not the lab work. Laboratory results can be misleading or nondiagnostic. In examining the patient, the physician must not be afraid to touch the patient to establish rapport. At the end of the visit, if the patient is agreeable, there's nothing wrong with a good hug to show affection and concern for the patient. Doctors should be honest with the patient and be willing to discuss all treatment options. There is usually more than one way to treat a given condition. As much as possible, the patient should be apprised of all the various treatment options and allowed to help make the decision as to which option they prefer. By doing so, the patient will be much more amenable and committed to the treatment program, increasing the chance for healing.

This is where faith comes in and may produce the placebo effect. Many doctors scoff at the placebo effect; however, it is a very powerful healing aspect to medicine and should not be ignored. Physicians take an oath to heal and not harm the patient. This should not be forgotten.

Patients are entitled to quality time and should not be rushed through the visit. A physician must explore the cause of the problem and not just treat the symptoms. Unfortunately, this is the focus of much of today's medicine. The symptoms are hastily treated by giving an allopathic drug and procedure without giving much thought to the possible side effects.

Independent studies report that fifteen to twenty-five percent of hospital admissions are because of medication side effects. I would like to refer you to the April 15, 1998, *Journal of the American Medical Association*. This publication notes that more than two million drug reactions occur yearly, killing more than one hundred thousand Americans and making prescription drugs the fourth leading cause of death in America. These figures relate only to those *properly prescribed drugs in the correct dosage*. I leave it to you to estimate the number of deaths and morbidity that have occurred because patients were given the incorrect drug combination or dosage. The pharmaceutical companies of America do not report these numbers. I strongly advise you to discuss your medications or other options with your doctor and have him tell you the possible side effects of the medicine. Always take as few prescription drugs as possible and stop taking the drugs as soon as possible.

Make no mistake; there are side effects from nutritional, herbal and other alternative therapies. However, the side effects from holistic therapies are less frequent and severe. The effectiveness of herbal therapy depends a great deal on where they are grown and in what type of soil. Because vegetables, fruit and herbs are reflective of the soil in which they grow, if the soil is deficient in a particular mineral, the crop will also be deficient. For instance, carrots grown in different places throughout the United States will have different compositions. Even though it looks like a carrot and tastes like a carrot, it will have major nutritional differences. It was recently reported that there are now some oranges that have little or no vitamin C. Also, because most herbs are dried, the positive effects of their essential aromatic oil properties have been eliminated.

The ability to listen to patients and keep an open mind has been very crucial and informative in my practice. Many of the alternative therapies I use today are the result of following a patient's suggestion to learn about a specific therapy. I am always ready, willing and able to try something new. I normally administer the suggested therapy to myself. If I think it might help a patient in some way and not cause a serious side effect, I prescribe the therapy to my patient. An elderly "traditional" physician once told me, "You young whippersnapper! I've been practicing medicine for almost fifty years. I don't think there's anything new to learn." I couldn't help replying to my friend, "Doctor, I disagree with you. I don't think you've been practicing medicine for almost fifty years." He looked startled. "Instead, I think you've been practicing one year of medicine fifty times." I think any doctor who is not willing to learn new techniques or new philosophies is probably doing the same thing over and over.

On another occasion, a friend and colleague gave me some fatherly advice about getting more rest. He suggested I was "burning the candles at both ends." I said, "Doctor, don't tell me that; just tell me where to get more wax." We had a good relationship, but sadly, the good doctor has now passed on. His methods of treating would not be adequate today nor would his record keeping. You see, he never kept a chart on a patient. Everything was kept in his head. I'm not sure how he remembered each patient's problem and medications. Somehow he managed. It certainly would not be acceptable today with all the emphasis on record keeping, lawsuits and malpractice insurance.

The practice of medicine has changed dramatically. It used to be joyful. Most doctors will agree that the past fifteen or twenty years have been plagued by government intervention, insurance regulations and legal reprisals. My solution has been to devote more energy to alternative, holistic, preventive, complementary and integrative medicine. Practicing in this manner has made medicine a rewarding profession again. I enjoy being a physician who, like a carpenter, has many tools in his toolbox.

Through the years, I have committed to memory a few sayings that are pertinent to life in general, and good health in particular. Alcoholics Anonymous advises its members to "live life day by day." This is very good advice. Since 1951 I have subscribed to another motto that says it just a little bit better, "Life is hard by the yard, but by the inch it's a cinch." I find many people live in the past instead of living in the now and looking forward to the future. I tell patients who live in the past to try to live their lives the way they drive a car. They should spend most of the time looking out the front windshield and only occasionally glancing in the rearview mirror.

It's better to wear out than rust out! Too often people retire, become couch potatoes and die prematurely. It is very important to keep active physically and mentally. Life is change and when you quit changing, you die, but to do this requires an active inquiring mind. In addition to a lack of exercise, improper eating habits and pollution, the worst factor facing us today is stress. Stress affects all illnesses and is difficult to combat. It comes in many forms: family problems, problems with friends, finances and even the government. Need I go on? There are several ways of combating stress. A simple one is to retreat to a private inner place. This inner place is within each of us and is easily reached once we learn how.

All of us have been collecting guideposts to this inner place, sometimes without realizing it. These guideposts or experiences help us feel calm and at peace with the world. These experiences include feelings, thoughts, and images of certain things like a beautiful sunset, fishing on a beautiful lake or relaxing in the sun at the seaside. Any calming experience can provide peace and security. When you feel stressed, reflect on these experiences. This practice will help you become relaxed and calm. Think of moments when you were caught up with the beauty around you. It might even be a color, the patter of rain on a roof, or a special song. Whatever it is, you've experienced many of these moments throughout your life. By paying attention to these memories, you can relieve the stress you are experiencing. This helps bring your body back to a state of balance.

Another way to combat stress is to avoid being judgmental. Everything has a good side and a bad side. If you try to look for the good in every circumstance, you will be less stressed and find most problems can be a source of enlightenment. Be optimistic. I am reminded of the old story about a boy who was punished by being placed in a large room full of horse manure. When his parents went back to check on him, they found him happily digging around in the horse manure. When asked why, he replied, "With that much horse manure, there must be a horse in there somewhere."

I use a stress management technique I've found extremely beneficial. I mentally place a screen around me. You can visualize a net, or as I do, a Polaroid screen totally encircling your body. As I envision it, this screen only allows the good to come through and reflects the bad. Therefore, while I am aware of the bad things in the world, I do not let them come in and affect me. Practice this mental exercise. To help you erect your barrier, sit with a lighted candle in a darkened room and visualize your screen.

Reducing stress can also be accomplished through the use of self-hypnosis, which is sometimes called autosuggestion. By progressive relaxation you can become relatively stress free, and give yourself positive suggestions to help in other aspects of daily life. Nothing is all bad or all good. If you look at the positive aspects of living, you will feel better, be healthier, and live longer more happily.

Another slogan I'm fond of is: "Take a stand and make a mark." If I feel very strongly about a subject, I will take a position and, despite all opposition, remain committed. I have adhered to this philosophy in my life as well as my profession. For example, I believe the Internal Revenue Service tax code is completely unconstitutional. For fourteen years I studied constitutional law and fought the IRS. They eventually took me to court on criminal charges and a jury agreed with my position, acquitting me.

I take the same zeal and determination into the realm of medicine. The reason I am writing this book is to acquaint you, a deserving and inquisitive public, with other approaches than the allopathic method of healing. I practice allopathic medicine every day and find it both helpful and necessary. But there are times when allopathic medicine does not provide the best answer. Using an alternative, holistic, complementary, integrative approach works better. These options should be available to everyone. I hope to persuade you not to fear these nonallopathic therapies and to discuss these approaches with your physician. I am doing all I can to build a bridge between allopathic and alternative forms of medicine.

Alternative, integrated medicine is not quackery. I deeply resent any doctor who denigrates these methodologies without investigating them. I get very upset when I hear physicians denouncing something about which they know nothing or that they have not tried. Physicians have to be open-minded and willing to listen. It is important not to jump to conclusions that are not based on fact and experience. If a physician researches alternative methods of healing and concludes it would not be helpful in his hands, I have no problem with his speaking against it.

When I hear professionals knock alternative medicine, I wish they would recall the old saying: "If you can't say something good, it's better to say nothing at all." Without really exploring the subject thoroughly, some narrow-minded professionals take an unyielding stand toward change. If they have experience and knowledge about the subject matter and believe it does not have value, then I respect their opinions.

I've said it before and I'll say it again—there are some life lessons we must learn. Live life day by day, live it by the inch…not by the yard. *Learn not to judge. Learn to love everyone, especially ourselves. You don't have to love what the person does, but love the person. Learn to forgive, especially yourself.* Thank God not only for the good things in our lives, but also for the bad things. This can be a troubling concept; however, if you keep an open mind, you can learn from both. What is one man's dessert may be another man's poison. *Never is a word to be avoided except in one instance. Never use the word hate. The word hate is one of the most destructive words in our vocabulary.*

Progress in life is like walking up stairs. As you take one step up, you have to leave one behind. You cannot go forward without leaving something behind. We progress at our own pace. We are all different. We should recognize the beauty in all things and deeply appreciate it. We continue to change throughout our entire lives. Therefore, your ideas on therapy should change as well. Try to improve yourself with each step you take forward. Eat better, exercise more, think positive thoughts and love yourself and your fellow man. Being healthy starts with thinking healthy. Avoid the negative pitfalls that so frequently assail us. Be open to new information, ideas and treatment programs.

Some of these might be very simple and inexpensive, so much so they are often not even considered. Just because it's simple and inexpensive does not mean it isn't good. For example, you can often get rid of warts by just taping a piece of the inner bark of a birch tree to the area. A toenail fungus often responds to applications of Vicks Vapor Rub or soaking your feet in your own urine. A simple inexpensive therapy for leg ulcers is the application of red wine compresses. Positive results are experienced in most instances.

We have to keep the cost of medicine under control. Anytime we can treat an illness with a safe and inexpensive method, we should do so without relying on the more expensive therapies. Let me give you an example: I treated an elderly diabetic gentleman who had previously had one leg amputated. He had had a stroke and developed advanced circulatory problems in his remaining leg. Following the amputation of his second leg, he developed gas gangrene in the stump. He was seen by numerous specialists and treated with thousands of dollars of the strongest antibiotics, all to no avail. After the specialists gave up hope and stopped the antibiotic therapy, I packed the stump in activated charcoal and directed a stream of oxygen against the stump. Within a week he showed marked improvement and eventually recovered. The specialists were truly amazed. More importantl, his life was saved for a few dollars a day and not the thousands that were being spent without success.

We are spending a great deal of money on cancer research, of which, until recently, much has been wasted. Billions of dollars have been spent in the past thirty plus years, with virtually no change in the outcome of this dreaded disease. Gene research shows promise. I envision immune stimulus, not destructive radiation and chemicals, as a likely answer. We need to continue medical research, but its focus must be redirected. Many research centers are now focusing on the immune system and genetic alteration. Science is finding many new medications and applications from natural sources, and research on new products from plants and trees shoulc be encouraged. Research on all the antioxidants is becoming popular. Investigation into human growth hormone and other therapies can give us additional longevity. Recently I read of a natural tree-based product that had an amazing effect on treating cancer. A pharmaceutical company tried in vain to make a drug out of it without success. When they couldn't develop it to make a profit, they abandoned it but did not inform the public that a natural substance existed that could help many with their cancers.

With all the new research in longevity, we should remember this basic precept: If you don't use it you'll lose it. I am also reminded of the saying: The way to stay young is to associate with young people. The way to get old is to try to keep up with them. I enjoy younger people, but I also like to associate with and treat older people. I find them to be full of wisdom gained through experience. The way to get the requisite experience is by living longer and healthier.

Since I do a lot of geriatric medicine, I am of the opinion everyone should be treated aggressively regardless of his or her age. I believe the only time people should not be treated actively is when their mental conditions are such that they are out of touch with reality, as in advanced Alzheimer's disease. Many doctors refuse to aggressively treat older patients because of their age. I am inclined to think this is utter nonsense. I treat eighty-or ninety-year old patients just as aggressively as twenty-year-olds if they have intact mental capacities. The success in treating any patient is not measured by populations, probability or popularity. It is measured by whether or not the individual believes that he or she is doing better. The focus on the individual is the beauty and strength of alternative medicine.

Alternative medicine is also described as complementary, and integrative. These terms apply equally, however; I prefer the term holistic. By holistic I mean, treating the whole person. Holistic medicine addresses the entire patient, not just the symptoms. Attention is paid to the physical, emotional and spiritual aspects of the patient because all are important whether you are two or one hundred and two years old. In practicing holistic medicine, I am preventing as well as treating illness. The patient and his physician work together to construct a therapy program. Therefore, it is not a dictatorial approach.

Most allopathic physicians do not take enough time with their patients and, consequently, they treat the symptoms without becoming knowledgeable about their patients. Time spent with the patient is critical to the prevention or elimination of any illness. When I see a patient, I perform a complete history and physical examination. Often, the most serious problem is not the one a patient presents. If the time is not taken, or the examination is not complete, a potentially serious problem can be overlooked. This may result in a crucial delay in treatment. Just as we were admonished as young children when learning to cross the street, I think doctors today should stop, look and listen more carefully to their patients. Even by doing so, we still have problems with difficult cases.

No matter the good intentions, physicians are still being pressured on all sides by their peers to stay faithful to the ideology they were taught in medical school. Medicine is influenced by patients who are ready to sue, and by insurance companies who will not cover all available treatment options. Health maintenance organizations (HMOs), preferred provider prganizations (PPOs) and Medicare regulate the types of treatment they will allow their patients to receive. As of July 1, 1998, a Medicare patient being treated by a Medicare physician is limited to the treatment programs Medicare approves. A patient must pay out of his own pocket for any other treatment he wants. Physicians are being forced to practice by the regulator's book, and the result is that physicians are being assaulted on all sides. Practicing traditional medicine isn't much fun.

I want to emphasize that I have not discarded allopathic medicine. There has been untold healing and care provided by allopathic drugs and therapy. There are countless capable allopathic physicians. I would like this book to be thought of as a bridge of new therapies to allopathic and alternative medicine, and better yet, as an expanded review of all methodologies.

Another fault of allopathic medicine is the overuse of antibiotics, which is causing numerous strains of bacteria to be resistant. Over one half of hospital staph infections are resistant to all types of antibiotics. The next several years will be critical in eliminating infections because of the resistant strains and the emergence of new and old diseases. It's important we continue using allopathic techniques; however, we must recognize that there is much more to medicine than curing illnesses with the allopathic therapies. New drugs and remedies will help build the body's immune system, but we have to learn to help ourselves with nature and its products.

It is a widely held belief in natural medicine that the Creator put all cures for illness in the plants of our earth. All we have to do is learn how to extract and apply them. It's more than just taking medicines, nutritional supplements, herbs or homeopathic remedies. I contend that the primary element is positive thinking. Starting with ourselves, we have to love and forgive everyone. And we have to learn not to judge. These are the very basic principles to which humankind must return to prevent most misery and suffering.

The other day I had a case that made me laugh. I was telling a new cancer patient he had to love and forgive and not to judge. His daughter, who brought him in, started laughing. When I asked her why, she said, "Do you know what my father's occupation is?" I said, "No, I don't." She replied, "He is a judge!" I laughed as well, and I asked him if he would consider giving up his occupation for a few months so we could build up his immune system and get the cancer under control.

I operated on a lady who had ovarian cancer. Her abdomen was totally studded with ovarian metastases. She had a large mass in her lower abdomen that was the primary source, or site, of the cancer. We removed the majority of the tumor. Even after we operated on her, she was so full of ovarian metastases throughout her abdomen that we did not expect her to live. I explained the situation to her husband postoperatively, but we never did tell the lady the extent of her cancer.

In an effort to decide how best to treat her, I called the Cleveland Clinic, University of Michigan, Mayo Clinic, Marshfield Clinic and Duluth Clinic. I was surprised to find everyone gave a different suggestion on how to treat her. I explained to the patient and her husband the treatment options offered by the different centers. I also told them that if they decided to stay with me, I would have a different way of treating her. At first she elected to go to the Mayo Clinic, but then changed her mind and decided to stay and be treated at home. I instituted a very unorthodox form of treatment. I adjusted her diet, put her on nutritional supplements and taught her mental imagery. With imagery, the patient visualizes her immune cells fighting the cancer cells and winning. We had the patient do this for five to ten minutes several times a day. I advised her to obtain both radiation and chemotherapy along with the nutritional therapy, and she survived.

I presented her case to a number of cancer clinics. Each suggested that I had given her excess chemotherapy and that she would probably develop leukemia sometime in the future. I disagreed because of the protective effects of the nutritional supplements. She did very well. Her only significant problem was the tendency to gain weight. I followed her case for twenty years, and she had no residual sign of cancer or leukemia. She eventually died of heart failure after I left Michigan. However, she lived twenty years longer than anyone expected.

A doctor should never absolutely predict how long a patient is going to live. Even though they may be trying to help the patient prepare for death, I think such limits are wrong for suggestible patients. Such patients tend to live for about the length of time others have predicted.

How long a person can live brings to mind another cancer patient. A Finnish lady had previously found a breast lump and was advised to have surgery. Finally, a year after the lump was discovered she agreed to have a mastectomy. She did very well postoperatively. Several years later, she presented with a lump on her back. My physician assistant thought it was an abscess and treated her with antibiotics for a week. It didn't show any improvement, so he had me look at it. We biopsied it and found it to be a metastatic lesion of her previous breast cancer. The chest X-ray showed she was full of metastatic lesions. Both lung fields were full of cancer. I had grave doubts as to how long she would survive. Had I been forced to make a guess it would have been several months. I showed her the X-ray and explained the findings. She expressed a desire to visit Finland. I told her to go to Finland to fulfill her wish. To improve her resistance I suggested she take twelve grams of vitamin C a day to help her strengthen her immune system. She agreed to this condition. I gave her a hug, wished her the best and said good-bye as she and her husband left the office.

When she walked into my office a year later I was totally flabbergasted. I was sure she would be dead by now. She looked great! I took a follow-up chest X-ray and it was completely clear. I'm not sure what caused the healing, but I'm sure the vitamin C played a role. When this lady discovered her lungs were clear and she was doing well, she inappropriately stopped her vitamin C therapy. A year later she developed skin cancer and eventually died from other causes.

Heart disease is one of the easiest illnesses to treat nutritionally. The heart is very receptive to nutritional therapy, especially a combination of garlic to reduce clotting and cholesterol; vitamin E to improve oxygenation and help dissolve small blood clots and magnesium to control heart rhythm. Taken in adequate doses, I can't recall any of my patients having had a heart attack or stroke on this program in the last ten years.

A number of arrhythmia's are caused by B-vitamin deficiencies. COQ-10 has been found to be beneficial to many people with heart failure. Standard Process and Biotics Research each make a multivitamin supplement that is very beneficial for strengthening the heart muscle and preventing arrhythmia. I have found, primarily in older women complaining of fatigue, that their problem is actually subclinical heart failure. They show marked improvement within several weeks of receiving multivitamins designed to strengthen the heart.

Standard Process and Biotics Research also each make a multivitamin to help diabetics lower blood sugars and eliminate large blood sugar swings. I have found these to be very beneficial for people who want to reduce or eliminate medications. Chromium can also be very effective in controlling diabetes as well as vanadium for diabetics with both high and low blood sugar. These should be dosed according to individual needs and not given haphazardly.

Everyone's chemistry is unique and if an herb, vitamin or mineral is good for one person it doesn't mean it's good for another. I cannot emphasize too often that there is a big difference in products made and labeled under various brands. Ginkgo biloba from one manufacturer may test very well for one patient, but another brand may not. Some doctors recommend a person take a standard amount of vitamin E, vitamin C and magnesium a day. Although the doctor's intentions are good, I believe this is misleading. Expensive testing methods can determine trace amounts of minerals and various vitamins. Patients can have treatment doses adjusted and a great deal of money can be saved if doctors would learn to treat via kinesiology.

Infections can be successfully treated with alternative, complementary methods. Oftentimes antibiotics do not have to be used in all cases. There are a number of immune activating products including herbs, vitamins and minerals on the market. Colloidal silver is a very good anti-infectant, and it has been found useful in bacterial as well as viral conditions. Compounds found in colostrum have also proven very beneficial in building the immune system. Infections and some forms of cancer have shown positive responses. NSC-24 (Beta-1, 3/1,6-glucan) is very effective. I have had a number of cases of various infections such as strep throat, sinusitis and pneumonia that did not respond to antibiotics but cleared up with NSC-24 without side effects.

The following examples illustrate NSC-24's potential:

- A patient had pneumonia for over two weeks and was not responding to several prescribed antibiotics, but after treatment with NSC-24 the infection cleared in one week.

- A second patient had a severe left maxillary sinusitis and had been on various antibiotics for six weeks. She was scheduled for sinus surgery but was afraid to have the procedure. She came to me hoping to find an alternate therapy. She did not test for any antibiotics that I kept on hand in my office. She was started on NSC-24, six times a day, and in seven days her symptoms were completely gone and her sinus X-ray was clear.

Two other products I have found that are very helpful are transfer factor and MSN-3. Transfer factor is especially good for infections and MSN-3 for treatment of cancer.

Nutritional supplements can help improve cataracts, glaucoma, headaches and leg cramps. The list is endless. Compared to prescription drugs, most of these nutritional supplements are not likely to cause any serious side effects and can be purchased without going into bankruptcy.

Everything changes. We must remember that although allopathic procedures are good and very well used, the theory that everything is right when proved by double-blind studies is not completely true. There have been numerous helpful medications and remedies used throughout the years that were not officially sanctioned by the double-blind process, for example, penicillin and the use of vitamin C for scurvy. Interestingly, cortisone was shown to be ineffective in a double-blind study, but it is still used frequently. Some medications and techniques do not fit the criteria for double blind studies such as acupuncture, aromatherapy and many massage techniques.

The most important aspect of healing is attitude, closely followed by nutrition. Proper breathing and exercise play vital roles. Willpower is also a determining factor in achieving good health. You have to believe. This will give you the best results in the shortest amount of time. I emphasize these to each patient I treat. I want my patients to be more healthy and less ill. I want patients to concentrate on preventing illness rather than treating an illness. I want patients to be responsible for their health. I expect patients to know what they are taking and why. I teach patients how to perform kinesiology so they can monitor their own medications. It would be my fondest wish to teach all medical doctors the use of kinesiology. It would greatly facilitate their practice of medicine. If nothing else, it would significantly diminish the number of side effects prescription medications often produce.

Most of us, especially in the medical profession, have received an education that has been too rigid and academic. We are attached to what we already know and ignore those things we don't understand. Many physicians believe that if they aren't knowledgeable about a subject, it probably doesn't exist. This belief must be given up.

Thomas Edison is well remembered for his work in the field of energy. He once stated, "The doctor of the future will give no medicine, but will interest his patients in the care of the human frame, in diet, and in the prevention of disease." Was he foreseeing alternative medical methods of chiropractic, Rolfing, myofacial release, nutritional therapy and energy medicine? Long before Dr. Edison, the Bible records in Mark 16:17–18, "And those signs shall follow them that believe in my name, they shall lay hands on the sick and they shall recover." This is being done today with health touch and reike. Both of these therapies are examples of energy medicine.

Those of us who are more concerned with prevention and healing rather than making a lot of money are investigating alternative therapies. We realize allopathic procedures and medication do not always provide adequate treatment for a myriad of current medical problems such as cancer, heart disease, hepatitis, viral infections, arthritis and so forth. However, there are alternative medical methods that have shown good results in addressing all of these illnesses. When I speak of alternative medical methods, I am referring to those not generally accepted by the allopathic community.

We need to bridge the gap between alternative and allopathic medicine. Physicians need to work together for the benefit of the patients and not remain attached to treatments that cover up the symptoms rather than provide a cure. In many cases, allopathic treatment has resulted in increased morbidity and higher medical costs.

I was a member of the American Medical Association for a number of years until I realized the AMA was not in agreement with my ideas for providing medical care. For example, we are told the AMA and the American Cancer Society are doing everything in their power to find the cause of cancer. They are actually also doing everything in their power to prevent physicians from using effective cancer cures presently available to them.

I had a personal experience regarding the treatment of skin cancer. I used an herbal salve to eliminate most common forms of skin cancer. With one or two applications I was successful over ninety-nine percent of the time. I rarely charged for this inexpensive solution. In spite of its excellent results, the Arizona Medical Board has forbidden me to use this product. If I practice what I know to be proper medicine, I will lose my medical license. I tried to get dermatologists in Phoenix and the dermatology department of the medical school at the University of California, Los Angeles (UCLA) to experiment with the salve. The secretary of the dermatology department of UCLA was very excited about the possibilities, but she was very dejected when she called me back and said they were not interested in testing the salve. Had they found out how well it worked, they would have had to consider giving up their surgical procedures.

Any doctor who finds an effective cancer treatment runs the risk of losing his license, being thrown in jail, harassed by the courts, or perhaps being driven out of the country, as a number of my acquaintances have been. The reason is money. The AMA is largely composed of professionals who believe healing can be achieved only through the use of prescription drugs and invasive surgery. The drug companies have been responsible for researching and developing many life saving and symptom reducing drugs. They are also partially responsible for brainwashing many medical practitioners. As increasing numbers of patients demand alternative therapies, more physicians are doing the research. Some doctors have taken off the blinders and have started experimenting with effective, alternative therapies.

Many doctors refuse to expand their treatment regimens for a number of reasons. Some believe double blind studies have to be performed to determine the effectiveness of any medication. Other doctors hesitate to use therapies because of peer pressure. Far too many physicians resist trying alternative methods because they are comfortable in crowds and resist thinking for themselves. They prefer to maintain tunnel vision, refusing to make the effort to research and try new methods. Most prefer to denounce and ridicule alternative therapies without taking the time or effort to find out how these alternative treatments perform.

Physicians should be among the leaders encouraging freethinking so that the greatest good could be achieved in treating the ills of the world. Favorable results, not the domination of one healing art over another, should be the goal. America has the best health care in the world, yet is one of the sickest nations because we have more chronic disease than many others.

Despite the fact we have more hospitals and medical schools, we have a long way to go to get to where we should be. It is becoming evident that hospitals should be avoided whenever possible because of drug-resistant strains of bacteria that are being encountered. Through the use of alternative care, I have been able to reduce my hospital admissions from an average of one to four a day to less than three a year. Imagine the amount of money saved by both patient and insurance companies.

"The art of medicine consists of amusing the patient while nature cures the disease."

Voltaire.

Chapter 3

The Body

The body is a wonderfully complex creation. At its best, the organs, glands, muscles and tissue work in a healthy harmony. The body's electronics, the nervous system, must smoothly carry energy to all systems! There can't be any shorts in the circuit. The body needs proper nutrition to function at peak performance. Natural food is the body's most efficient fuel. Natural foods will supply more health-giving nutrition than artfully processed foods. However, no food will keep the machine running if the digestive system is not properly assimilating the nutrition.

Amazing Facts About Your Body

- Except for brain cells, fifty million of the cells in your body will have died and been replaced by others all while you have been reading this sentence.

- The adult heart beats about forty million times a year. In one hour the heart works hard enough to produce enough energy to raise almost one ton of weight one yard off the ground. It pumps six quarts of blood through ninety-six thousand miles of blood vessels.

- The liver is often called the body's chemical factory. Scientists have counted over five hundred different liver functions.

- Forty-three pairs of nerves connect the central nervous system to every part of the body. Twelve pairs go to and from the brain and thirty-one pairs go to and from the spinal cord. There are nearly forty-five miles of nerves running through our bodies.

- Messages travel along the nerves as electrical impulses. The fastest they travel is about 248 miles per hour.

- In one square inch of skin there are four yards of nerve fibers, thirteen hundred nerve cells, one hundred sweat glands, three million cells and three yards of blood vessels.

- The brain has twenty-five billion cells.

- The skin has four million pores for cooling and eliminating.

- The body has seventy-five trillion cells all working together. Each cell has more chemical reactions than all the chemical factories in the world! Between three hundred billion and eight hundred billion cells are replaced every day.

- In much less than one year all of the cells in your body except the brain have been replaced by new cells; for example, red blood cells are replaced every 120 days. Therefore, with proper thinking and correct nutrition, the new cells can be manufactured by the body to be better and healthier than the old ones they replaced. Just think of that—a new body in less than one year.

- Rebuilding your body is a lot like building a new house. You want to eat the best food, that is, natural, fresh and free from chemicals—just like you want the best building materials so your house will last a long time. You want to think properly and positively just as you would want a good architect and carpenters to do.

Water

Over seventy percent of the body is water. More than ninety percent of our brain is water. Water is more important to your health than food. You can live many days without food, but not water. Of the world's water, ninety-seven percent is held in the oceans, unfit for drinking; two percent of the planet's water is frozen in the ice caps, leaving only one percent readily available for drinking. How much of this one percent is uncontaminated? I'm certain our drinking water is more polluted than anyone imagines. Don't rely on your public water source. Most public water supplies are purified with chlorine. It is your responsibility to assure the water you use is safe. It needs to be free of chlorine that can cause allergies and respiratory problems. It may contribute to arteriosclerosis. Research has indicated it may also increase risk of bladder and rectal cancer.

Remember, you absorb more chlorine by far from showering with chlorinated water than by drinking it.

Another main problem is that most water we drink is fluoridated. As a chemistry major in college I learned that fluoride was one of the most dangerous chemicals known to man. Even a small mistake in the amount of fluoride added to the water supply or to our toothpaste can be exceedingly dangerous. I have recently been informed that *contaminated fluoride,* which has contained toxic lead, arsenic and radium, has been dumped into our water supplies for years. In addition to the potential cancer threat from these toxic minerals, the fluoride is also causing dental fluorosis and skeletal abnormalities. Avoid fluoride more than you should avoid chlorine.

Another toxic chemical in this group is bromine. The only other chemical in this group is iodine, which in large amounts is also dangerous. However, in many persons we find a deficiency that is much less now that table salt has had iodine added. By the way, I also don't recommend you eat table salt, since it has been adulterated too much. Instead I recommend you use a good sea salt—the brand I prefer is Real Salt, which can be obtained from most health food stores.

Tap water should be filtered before drinking. There are many good water purifiers and distillers on the market. If you use a distiller, be sure to use multiple mineral supplements. All municipal water supplies are susceptible to contamination from multiple infectious and chemical agents including chlorine poisoning. It has been estimated that more than twelve hundred people die each year in the United States from drinking contaminated tap water. Consider then the number of deaths in the third world countries attributed to poor water quality. In 1993 an outbreak of cryptosporidiosis occurred in Milwaukee, Wisconsin. It was the largest waterborne disease outbreak ever to have occurred in the United States with an estimated four hundred thousand persons affected. There are many examples of pathogens that are known to be transmitted through contaminated water, such as the bacteria salmonella, shigella, campy lobacter, toxigenic E coli, and heliobacter pyloric. There are also numerous protozoa and some viruses. Very few water treatment plants are able to maintain fully protected water sources. Air pollution and wild life can contaminate our watersheds as well as terrorists.

Water treatment has long depended on disinfections as the primary barrier. However, disinfections have come under scrutiny because of disinfection by-products that have been associated with increases in bladder and other cancers. Alternatives to chlorination such as ozone treatment are becoming popular.

Infectious disease is not the only problem. The ease of distribution of contaminated water makes outbreaks of chemical poisonings likely. A number of such outbreaks are reported to the Centers for Disease Control and Prevention each year. Arsenic, mercury and organic solvent poisoning related to geological or industrial contaminated ground water are common examples.

Not only is it important to your health to drink pure water, but you should also drink plenty of it! Recently, two epidemiologists from Loma Linda University in California reported that drinking five glasses of water a day was associated with significant decreased fatal coronary artery disease and a substantially lowered risk of fatal stroke. It has been my experience that increased water intake has positive effects on heartburn, fatigue, constipation, asthma attacks and healthy skin. It has even been helpful in reducing the problems associated with jet lag. The body needs a lot of water to function properly and aid in the elimination of waste products and toxins.

I am currently doing a research clinical study on water that has been structurally altered by passing through a series of pyramids of different sizes. So far it has shown a good deal of promise in treating a number of medical problems.

In future books I hope to have case studies and examples of my research in pyramid water therapy.

Update
It has been over one year since I wrote this chapter. I would like to update you on our water problems.

According to a California think tank, as many as seventy-six million people—mostly children—could die from water-related diseases by 2020 if changes aren't made worldwide. The United Nations says 1.1 billion people worldwide live without access to safe drinking water. More people die of diarrheic diseases such as dysentery than other water-related diseases, and children are extremely vulnerable to them. We are having a very dry year, especially those of us in the western states. Many are wondering if we are entering an era similar to the dust-bowl years. Many large forest fires have destroyed thousands of acres. (We have had several such fires here in Arizona.) Many wells are going dry. More and more people are drinking bottled water. I have tested many brands with kinesiology and find that some popular brands do not test well. You need to learn kinesiology so you can determine which brands to avoid.

We are in a giant multiyear drought that is spreading around the world. Once our most common resource, water is becoming one of our scarcest and most precious commodities. Our next major war may well be over water instead of oil. The *McAlvany Intelligence Advisor*—July 2002 issue—deals in detail with the world's water shortage that in turn will lead to worldwide food shortages.

In America we have multiple problems:

- The Environmental Protection Agency (EPA) stated in April 2002 that forty-four percent of the coastal waters were so polluted that they cannot sustain aquatic life, fishing or human activities.

- Human waste that contains toxic chemicals and pharmaceutical drugs is being discharged into rivers and lakes, causing much pollution and subsequent potential disease problems.

- Recycled water (chemically treated toilet water) is being used as drinking water by millions of Americans! How does that sound to you? To be safe don't drink any tap water in the United States.

- United States lakes, rivers and reservoirs are going dry, causing severe restrictions on irrigation needed for food production.

- Forest fires resulting from extra-dry conditions cause devastation to the woodlands and secondarily to the water sheds and rivers.

- The Colorado River, which supplies Arizona and California with much-needed water, is being mostly used up before it even reaches the ocean.

- Americans have to conserve what water we have and use it very wisely. You might want to consider investing in water because it is a very necessary product that is being depleted at a rapid rate.

- Water can be made available from desalinization of the ocean water and also from the melting of icebergs, but these methods are expensive and at present only supply a relatively small amount of drinking water.

Nutrition

In the United States we are overfed and undernourished, prompting numerous commercial diets from Atkins to Pritikin. There are diets based on blood type, gender, ethnic background and geographic location, to mention just a few. Many diets are diametrically opposed and at best can be described as fads. We must remember that diets, as well as supplementation, must be individualized.

There is no diet concept better than proper nutrition. Everyone is chemically different and in a constant state of change. Diets need to be individualized. A proper diet this year might need to be changed significantly next year. A diet should take into account the results of laboratory tests including fasting blood sugar, cholesterol level, triglycerides and liver/kidney functions. Natural food is the body's most efficient fuel. The body is always striving for health by continuously cleaning the gastrointestinal tract, kidneys, liver and skin. The subconscious controls all functions.

St. Patrick's Diet

We eat too much refined (manufactured) food and *simple* carbohydrates, including potatoes, rice, alcohol, bananas, figs and dates that quickly metabolize into sugar. We need to eat more *complex* carbohydrates and protein. I am a proponent of the nutritional principles found in what I like to call the St. Pat's diet. I obtained the diet from the St. Patricia's Healing Center in Minneapolis in 1969, making minor adjustments to the diet outline based on the patient's diagnosis. Natural foods will supply more health giving nutrition than artificially processed foods.

The following is my modified version of St. Patricia's Diet. I advise my patients that the *following foods are not good for their health and should be avoided wherever possible.*

Wheat Flour
Any food containing white flour such as bread, cookies, pies and cakes. Use whole wheat, rye, and so forth. Although I understand that breads made with whole wheat or rye contain some white flour, it is much better to eat these breads than the all white flour variety.

White Sugar
White sugar and foods made with white sugar, such as soft drinks, Jell-O, ice cream, and chocolate. Honey or stevia can be used as a sweetening substitute.

Hydrogenated Fats and Oils
Hydrogenated fats, oils, and solid cooking fats such as Crisco, reheated fats, animal fat and margarine. I recommend the use of virgin olive oil for cooking, however, butter is allowed. Canola oil is to be avoided.

Processed and Packaged Foods
Highly processed and packaged food often contains multiple preservatives, artificial colorings, flavors, emulsifiers, stabilizers, nitrates, sulfides and monosodium glutamate (MSG).

Pasteurized and Homogenized Milk
Pasteurized and homogenized milk. It is much better to use raw or skim cow's milk, goat's milk, soy or rice milk. Use pasteurized skim milk when no preferred products are available. Pasteurization makes milk safer; however, it alters the chemistry of the calcium and protein and renders the milk less beneficial to the body. All of the things being fed to cows today make their milk less desirable. Artificial hormones and chemicals can be very deleterious to your health. Unless you're a calf, you probably don't need milk! Homogenization is another process making fat globules so small they don't collect on the top of the milk bottle in a layer of fat. Unfortunately, these very small fat particles can pass directly into the blood stream through the gastrointestinal tract and lead to fat metabolism problems.

Fried Foods, Chips, White Rice and White Potatoes
Fried foods, chips, white rice and white potatoes should be limited. Brown rice and red potatoes are preferred. If you must use white potatoes, baking will make them more digestible.

Alcohol, Cocoa, Chocolate and Coffee
Alcohol, cocoa, chocolate, instant and regular coffee should also be used on a limited basis only. Alcohol should be avoided or limited to two ounces a day. This amount has actually been found to be beneficial.

Fish and Shellfish
Fish and shellfish including lobster, scallops, clams, oysters, shrimp, and so forth, can increase your triglyceride levels. While it is all right to eat these foods on an occasional basis, they should not be a regular part of any diet. Cold ocean fish have been found to contain toxic chemicals. Most of the chemicals are concentrated in the liver and lateral line (gray area along the outside of the fish under the skin). If you avoid eating these, your chances of eating excessive toxic chemicals are reduced.

Pork
Pork should be avoided for the most part because it is difficult to digest.

Salt
Excess salt intake. Most foods are oversalted to begin with. Some sea salt is acceptable. Sea salt, called Real Salt, tests best on most people. Red cayenne pepper is not only acceptable but can be very beneficial.

Canned Foods
Eliminate canned foods when frozen or fresh are available.

Since I recommend avoiding all of the above, what do I suggest you eat? There are a wide variety of healthful foods you can eat. Vegetables of all colors contain different carotenoids. These act to prevent cancer and stimulate the immune system. The most nutritious vegetables are asparagus, avocado, beets, broccoli, Brussels sprouts, cabbage, cauliflower, carrots, celery, cucumbers, egg plant, onions, peas, radishes, sauerkraut, squash, string beans, tomatoes, turnips, lettuce, mushrooms and raw nuts. Fresh green vegetable juice, carrot juice and beet juice are probably three of the most healthful juices you can drink.

To obtain the enzymes missing in cooked or processed foods, raw foods should make up the majority of your diet. The more raw foods you eat, the better. Contrary to traditional thinking, there is no limit to the number of eggs you can eat. At this point I'd like to share with you an *egg*ceptional story. I had a patient with a reported cholesterol count of *5000*. Yes, 5000! In my entire medical career, I've seen patients with cholesterol levels between 500/1000. My own cholesterol had once been as high as 1000. This patient, however, had the highest lipid level I had ever seen. Most of you will say a 5000 cholesterol count is impossible. I retested him at several different laboratories with similar results. I instructed him to go home, take several nutritional supplements, and eat all the eggs and butter he wanted. Within six months his cholesterol returned to normal.

I then sent him to the Mayo Clinic for an evaluation of his lipid chemistry. When he returned, he told me they had found nothing abnormal and that he should quit taking the nutritional supplements that I had advised. This upset me, so I called the doctor at the clinic and asked him for the reason why he had told the patient to quit following my advice. He said the things I had prescribed didn't work. Therefore, he saw no reason to continue them. I then asked him if he had ever used them or if he knew anything about the supplements I had advised. He answered that he did not know anything about them. I then suggested that since they did work very well and since he did not have anything specific against them, perhaps the patient should continue instead of stopping them. After a long thoughtful pause, the doctor stated he may have been wrong and that he would now advise the patient to continue. I think this is a good example—if a doctor doesn't already know about something—he thinks the probability of it being beneficial is unlikely!

For people with hypoglycemia, I alter the diet slightly. With hypoglycemia, I recommend eating small meals frequently and avoiding big meals. As with any other medical problem, there are all degrees of hypoglycemia from mild to severe. The more severe the problem, the stricter you will have to be with your diet. In addition to frequent meals, you have to avoid the starches, sugars and simple carbohydrates, which rapidly metabolize into starches and sugars.

The following foods are absolutely contraindicated in patients with severe hypoglycemia: alcohol, soft drinks, club soda, whiskey, liqueurs, sugar, candy, cakes, pies, pastries, sweet custards, puddings and ice cream. You should also be very judicious in your consumption of caffeine—coffee and tea. Potatoes, rice, grapes, raisins, plums, dates, figs and bananas should be avoided. Spaghetti, noodles, macaroni, jams, jellies and marmalades should also be avoided whenever possible. Any nonsweetened cranberry or vegetable juice, herb tea, decaffeinated coffee and coffee substitutes are allowable.

Many people have food allergies, which can cause a myriad of symptoms. The most common allergy-producing foods are eggs, yeast, wheat, milk, corn and soybeans. Every one of these foods is found in a wide variety of prepared products, which some you might not even be aware of. Contrary to popular belief, excess soy consumption has been reported to cause thyroid problems, sexual problems and autoimmune diseases.

A list of these hidden foods is included in the chapter entitled Food Allergies. Foods a person is allergic to should be avoided if at all possible. There are natural substances a person can take to minimize their reaction to foods. One is a form of the mineral molybdenum. Another is methylsulfonylmethane, otherwise known as MSM. Some people can have their food allergy symptoms decreased using a product from Biotics Research called Pneumazyme. An alternative therapy called Nambudripad's Allergy Elimination Technique (NAET) is very effective for eliminating all allergies (Devi S. Nambudripad, M.D. created the therapy).

Sensitivity to sulfides is quite common. Foods containing high levels of sulfides include commercial avocado dip, guacamole, dried fruits, dried and frozen potatoes, dehydrated vegetables, shrimp, wine products and vegetable bars in restaurants.

Another common chemical to which many people are sensitive is monosodium glutamate, or MSG. The FDA does not require MSG labeling on food products.

Therefore you must be aware of the sources of MSG and read the labels. The primary "hidden" sources of MSG are hydrolyzed protein, sodium casseinate, calcium casseinate, autolyzed yeast or yeast extract and gelatin. Other likely sources of MSG are tetraprotein, vegetable gum, carrageenan, seasonings, spices, flavorings, chicken, beef or pork bouillon, broth, barley, malt, malt extract, whey protein, whey protein isolate or concentrate and soy sauce.

Too many of my patients drink fluids with their meals. This habit dilutes the hydrochloric acid in the stomach, preventing proper digestion. Most people don't drink enough water. It is a good idea for most patients to drink half of their weight in ounces of water daily. For example, a person who weighs 170 pounds should drink eighty-five ounces daily. With some illnesses and in very dry climates, more may be needed. Clean water, in the proper amounts, is essential to achieving your nutritional goals. Most of our water supply is chlorinated or fluorinated. These elements create major health hazards because they replace the iodine in the body and lead to higher incidences of subclinical hypothyroidism. Fluoride and chlorine contribute to a less than effective immune system. Fluoride in anything but micro doses is toxic. More chlorine can be absorbed through the skin in a hot shower than by drinking chlorinated water. Evaluate the water you use and take the steps necessary to safeguard your health. There are numerous newsletters devoted exclusively to nutrition. Review those authored by Drs. Jonathan Wright, Julian Whitaker, Bruce West, David Williams, John J. Nugent or William Douglas and subscribe to the one(s) that interest you the most.

"You are what you eat and think"—Dr. Schroeder, et al.

Vitamins, Supplements and Herbs

More and more physicians advocate the use of vitamins. Antioxidants have been researched and proven valuable in the prevention and treatment of degenerative diseases and cancers. Doctors no longer dismiss vitamins simply as a cause of expensive urine. As with anything else, there are good vitamins and bad vitamins. It's important that you use *natural* vitamins. Natural *complexes* are even better, because they have other nutrients that enhance their performance. Synthetic vitamins are chemicals. We have far too many in our environment, as is evidenced by worldwide pollution. Pollution is present in the skies, soil, foods, and water supply. These chemical pollutants are a major factor in many illnesses. The number one priority of prevention therapy is the improvement of our immune status.

Synthetic vitamins are vitamins in name only. The term *vitamin* deceives the public. Synthetic vitamins can cause sickness and even death to unsuspecting people genuinely interested in improving their health. The manufacturers of these synthetic vitamins claim that their products have the same molecular structure and benefits of natural vitamins. They don't mention, however, that the polarity of the synthetic is usually opposite of the natural vitamin with the opposite effects.

Synthetic vitamins refract light in the opposite way of natural vitamin complexes. Dr. Royal Lee, the founder of the Standard Process Company, discovered the light refraction attributes of vitamins in the 1930's. He has subsequently developed many natural supplements, which I have used since 1969.

There are potent supplements such as melatonin, dehydroepiandosterone (DHEA) and human growth hormone (HGH) being taken without sufficient knowledge on the part of the consumer or health care practitioner. These supplements have specific applications in the treatment of certain illnesses; however, many of the doses are taken indiscriminately.

Consequently, there is a movement to have nutritional supplements supervised by a physician. I have three concerns about this:

- Most physicians are less educated on the benefits of nutritional supplements than their patients. This could lead the physician to lean toward something he knows, more allopathic medications.

- When physicians, inexperienced in nutritional therapy, recommend supplements they become liable for the management of any side effects.

- With physician involvement comes the next logical, legislative step; the need for a prescription to purchase vitamins/supplements. Without a doubt the prices for these items will skyrocket.

There are those who try to discredit the benefits of vitamin therapy by designing experiments intended to produce misleading results. For example, a 1994 Finnish study reported that beta-carotene was not helpful in treating lung cancer; in fact, the report claimed that it actually made cancers worse. It is important to note that the public was not informed that the study used the synthetic form of beta-carotene rather than the natural form. Was this done to intentionally mislead the public regarding the positive effects of vitamins? The Mayo Clinic undertook a study to determine the effect of vitamin C on the treatment of the common cold. They reported that vitamin C had no effect; however, the doses they used were far too small to be of benefit. I caution you to be skeptical about what you hear and read. Do your homework. Research the product. Seek the advice of your physician and insist on kinesiology testing of every nutritional supplement you ingest.

I've often been asked what vitamins and supplements I personally use. What I take is determined by kinesiology testing. The dosage varies with my metabolism and health. What I use in January might be completely different from what I use in April or September. Let me give you an example of my basic nutritional regimen by the numbers.

Vitamin E

Vitamin E was the first nutritional supplement I used. Vitamin E is thought to dissolve small blood clots and improve circulation and oxygenation. I have also found that it helps joint symptoms in selected cases. Starting in 1969 I have taken either 400 or 800 milligrams of *d-Alpha* vitamin E. The synthetic vitamin E, dl-alpha tocopherol, produces more side effects and complications and should be avoided. I sometimes take an emulsified form of vitamin E as well as a water-soluble vitamin E. I've had to quit taking vitamin E for one to three months due to test results that indicated I had enough vitamin E stored in my fatty tissues to sustain metabolic balance.

A snowmobile club I was associated with planned a trip from Marquette, Michigan to West Yellowstone National Park. I realized I'd be climbing to a much higher elevation than the one I was familiar with in Marquette. Also, I knew I'd require extra endurance to operate the machines in deep snow. Therefore, I increased my water-soluble vitamin E to 4,000 milligrams. Within a few weeks I developed a cardiac arrhythmia. My associate became concerned and referred me to the Cleveland Clinic for angiograms. The results were negative, however the cardiologist told me he was still concerned that something was wrong with my heart.

I suspected that the cardiac problem was related to the increased doses of vitamin E, but I was embarrassed to reveal my excesses. I subsequently decreased my vitamin E intake to 800 milligrams per day and my cardiac arrhythmia subsided. It is the only side effect of natural vitamin E I have seen in my practice. The moral of the story is that even too much of a good thing can be harmful.

I treated an elderly non-ambulatory gentleman with vitamin E while he was confined in the hospital. Within a week he was able to walk without difficulty. He received no other treatment to account for this improvement. I stopped his vitamin E as a trial, and within a few days he returned to his non-ambulatory status. I restarted his vitamin E, and he returned to his previous level of mobility. In this particular case, vitamin E had a remarkable effect on his muscle and joint symptoms.

I saw a young man in the emergency room who was badly burned over most of his body. His house had caught fire and he had gone back in to rescue his dog. In the process, he received severe burns on his chest, face, hands and arms. The doctors who saw him initially advised that he be transferred to a major burn center. His mother did not want him moved, so I volunteered to take charge of this case. In addition to using antibiotics and intravenous fluids he was treated primarily with topical and oral vitamin E.

His hands healed; however, due to the severity of his burns, he developed web-like scar tissue between the fingers. I performed cosmetic surgery to free up the adhesions; however, his face remained scarred from the burns. He came in one day quite depressed because the other children at school were calling him "Scarface." I hypnotized him and suggested that he should be very proud of his scars, and consider them a badge of honor to show his bravery in saving his pet. I further suggested that the other children's remarks would not bother him in the future. He continued to attend school with no further emotional episodes regarding the taunts of his classmates. I was very pleased at how well his scars were doing using vitamin E. They actually seemed soft and pliable compared to most burn scars. He allowed me to take a biopsy of the scar. We had the biopsy stained for elastic tissue and, surprisingly, found elastic tissue in the scar.

Two years later my young patient came into the office to say hello. I did not recognize him. His face was totally healed. There was no significant scarring. He was a very good-looking young man. I was amazed at how well he had healed thanks, in no small part, to vitamin E therapy. Recently a new form of vitamin E has become available. Much more powerful are tocotrienols, which are slightly different than alpha-tocopherol. They are up to sixty times more potent as an antioxidant and can also lower cholesterol and decrease blood clotting. They have no known side effects. One available source of tocotrienols is the brand name, Care Diem. It also inhibits Thromboxane A2, similar to aspirin, so I believe it would be of benefit as it doesn't cause any stomach irritation.

Another product, Pam Vitea, is a special tocotrienol preparation made from palm oil. It has been shown to decrease the likelihood of a second stroke by thinning the blood and dissolving arterial plaque.

Multivitamin/Multimineral Supplement

For most patients, a balanced foundation of multiple vitamins and minerals is essential. Please consider taking a good multiple vitamin, one that tests well for you as part of your nutritional program. Taking one vitamin or mineral to excess often leads to deficiencies in other vitamins and minerals. Balance is the key. Certain substances interact with others and cause difficulties with absorption, and so forth. For example, vitamin E and iron should not be taken together. Too much of one B vitamin can alter the balance of other B vitamins. Calcium interferes with zinc absorption. Because of the differences in our bodies, Biotic Research has six different multiple vitamin/mineral formulas to choose from to accommodate differences between male and female needs, diabetics, hypoglycemics, heart conditions and menopausal patients. The multiple vitamins contain three very important vitamins for heart health. Vitamin B_6, folic acid and B_{12} act together to keep your homocystean levels normal. Homocystene elevations tend to lead to heart disease and also possibly to Alzheimer's disease. Many multiple vitamins on the market do not have sufficient levels of these three vitamins. So be sure to read the labels. Most people require 800 micrograms of folic acid, 500 to 1,000 micrograms of vitamin B_{12} and 25 to 50 micrograms of vitamin B_6.

Vitamin C

Vitamin C has proven its worth over and again even in its synthetic form. Since man does not manufacture his own vitamin C, it must be included in his diet. High doses of vitamin C have been effective in treating some cancers, the common cold and most infections. Vitamin C can also enhance the immune system and help minimize atherosclerosis. I have had numerous allopathic physicians tell me that high doses of vitamin C are dangerous but I have not seen any evidence to support their opinion. On the contrary, Dr. Linus Pauling, a Nobel Prize winner, did extensive research on vitamin C and concluded that large doses of vitamin C actually improved the longevity of many cancer patients. Dr. Pauling personally took 10,000 milligrams or more of vitamin C a day.

It is widely known that smokers have more blood vessel disease than non-smokers. But did you know that each cigarette tends to deplete the vitamin C level by approximately fifty milligrams? A vitamin C supplement is essential for anyone foolish enough to smoke. There is a plausible theory that vitamin C deficiency gives symptoms similar to those of subclinical scurvy. The theory further contends that subclinical scurvy produces microhemorrhaging, especially in the blood vessels. Cholesterol then deposits over these bleeding sites like a scab on a wound. When this happens repeatedly over several months or years, there is a build-up of cholesterol plaque.

AntiOxidants

There are many nutritional antioxidants. I will give you a partial list of the more frequently used ones. In the recent past, the medical establishment has recognized antioxidants. There has been extensive medical research on the use of antioxidants, and a great deal of information is available in medical journals and magazines. You might think of antioxidants as anti-aging products that also help improve the immune system and help protect us from a variety of diseases, including cancer. Two of the most common antioxidants are vitamin E and vitamin C, however there are many others. I have found that each one has a specific effect on our immune system, while taken in combination, the antioxidants enhance the properties of each and provide a better result than when taken separately.

Pyconogenal is a relatively new antioxidant. It is produced from pine bark and/or grape seed extracts. Pycnogenol is alleged to have greater antioxidant activity than either vitamin E or vitamin C. Pyconogenol was the strongest antioxidant available until just recently. Microhydrin, a hydrogen ion substance, seems to have the greatest antioxidant effect of any known substance. Selenium, vitamin A, some of the B vitamins, some of the amino acids and some of the carotinoids are examples of other antioxidants.

In addition to the other antioxidants and multiple vitamins, I also take an antioxidant product from Biotic Research called BioProtect. It is a combination of vitamin A, vitamin E, vitamin C, Selenium, co-enzyme Q-10, Sorbic acid, glutathione, L-methionine, taurine, N-acetyl-L-cysteine, zinc, superoxide dismutase and catalase.

In my opinion, anyone wanting to live healthier and longer must take adequate amount of antioxidants. Once again, each person should be tested individually for the most effective antioxidants and the proper dose of each.

Organic Flaxseed Oil

Prior to flaxseed oil I used fish oil. Fish oil is very beneficial for certain types of arthritis, mild blood pressure problems and some cardiac arrhythmias. Fish oil tends to lower cholesterol and influence the clotting mechanisms so that blood does not easily clot. Dry skin and dry hair can also be improved.

Michigan State University did a study on fish from all waters of the world and found that various chemicals such as DDT and dioxines contaminated all species. Since fish oil comes primarily from the liver, I felt there was a danger of chemical contamination. Consequently, I changed to organic flax oil. Both fish oil and organic flax oil contain Omega 3 and Omega 6, fatty acids that are good for our body.

I recommend only chemically free organic flax oil. Women, especially, should take organic flax oil for the prevention of breast cancer. Recently the Tyler Company produced a fish oil capsule, which it claims is free of toxic chemicals. I have tested it and find it acceptable and therefore now use both flax and fish oil in selected patients.

Magnesium/Calcium

Most people in this country are more deficient in magnesium than calcium. The three most common symptoms of magnesium deficiency I see in my office are emotional, (depression and irritability) constipation and cardiac arrhythmia. Of course, there are many other conditions where magnesium will benefit a patient, such as enlargement of the prostate and male infertility. Magnesium is the most critical mineral required for the proper regulation of our electrical system.

A calcium-magnesium compound provides the best supplement. The ratio of calcium to magnesium is open for discussion. Some researchers suggest two parts calcium to one part magnesium and others suggest the opposite. I generally recommend that my patients use more magnesium than calcium. In fact, I take an additional magnesium supplement because it is vital to many chemical reactions in our body. Almost every illness has been found to be accompanied by low magnesium levels.

Rubidium

Rubidium is not yet considered one of the essential trace elements, but several clinical studies have shown that rubidium has a special role in the transport of minerals across cell membranes, especially the membranes of cells damaged by normal aging. Rubidium transports iodine into the thyroid and is sometimes useful in treating thyroid conditions. There is also some indication that rubidium attaches itself to the cancer cell membrane and helps neutralize toxic enzymes, leading to the death of the cancer cell. This theory is supported by the fact that in geographic areas where diets are high in rubidium, the incidence of cancer is very low. I take rubidium because it has been shown to reduce memory loss associated with aging. Now that I am in my late sixties, I feel that I need all the help I can get.

Colostrum

Mother's milk is one of nature's finest and most perfect combinations of immune factors. It is life's first food and has tremendous potential throughout our lifetime. It has been found to be useful in helping to rebuild the immune system, along with fighting acute viral and bacterial infections. Colostrum has also been found useful in the treatment of some cancers and allergies. I have been treating patients with colostrum for about five years and have been very impressed with the results. Colostrum contains growth factors that help build lean muscle tissue and burns fat for energy, thereby aiding weight loss. It also contributes to building and repairing RNA and DNA as well as increasing protein synthesis.

At present, bovine colostrum has been shown to be completely safe, with no drug interactions or side effects at any dosage level. Colostrum is another natural agent we can use against the "super bugs" that are highly resistant to many of today's antibiotics. There are a number of products available that contain colostrum.

Garlic

Garlic is my favorite herb. If I had to give up all supplements except one, I'd keep garlic. Garlic contains many minerals and is very supportive of the immune system. Garlic has a very powerful anti-parasitic and anti-infectious component. I instruct all my patients who travel to Mexico to take an ample dose of garlic every day. Garlic has been found to reduce the fibrinogen level in your blood and helps prevent excess blood clotting. Thus helping to prevent strokes and heart attacks. Garlic, magnesium and vitamin E are the "Big Three" supplements in preventing cardiovascular problems. The dosage depends on periodic testing by kinesiology.

Ginkgo Biloba

Ginkgo Biloba is an herb shown to improve circulation for the heart, brain and prostate. It also enhances the memory.

Chromium

I take chromium intermittently depending on my HDL levels of cholesterol. I also use it for episodes of hypoglycemia.

Niacinacol

This is a non-flushing form of niacin aiding in the control of cholesterol levels. I use niacinacol periodically because my cholesterol levels tend to be normal to slightly elevated. My cholesterol levels are tremendously improved compared to my college years, when they were over 1,000. In addition to Niacinacol, there are a multitude of natural therapies that are shown to effect cholesterol levels. Natural anti-cholesterol agents include garlic, lethicin, vitamin C, calcium, a high-fiber diet, L-cartinine, niacin, the Omega-3 and Omega-6 oils, alfalfa, pectin, egg plant, inositol, methionine, choline, some vegetable oils, vitamin B-6, magnesium, L-Arginine, L-Cysteine and L-Carnitine. I rarely recommend any of the allopathic drugs for elevated cholesterol due to their many side effects.

There are five other nutritional supplements I have begun to evaluate over the past two years. They are MSM (methysulfonylmethane), NSC-24, MGN-3, Transfer Factor and Microhydrin. MSM is a natural sulfur compound found in all living things. It is no less important to your diet than vitamin C. MSM is also another antioxidant that helps detoxify the body. MSM has also been found to improve athletic performance and tends to be a tremendous energy booster. MSM plays many roles in the body, including the stimulation of growth of healthy skin, hair and nails. It is needed to produce healthy connective tissue, proper enzyme activity and hormonal balance, along with the proper function of the immune system. As a sulfur compound, MSM is one of the building blocks of amino acids. MSM works best when taken with vitamin C; together, they build healthy new cells. MSM provides bonding between the cells and increases the flexibility of cells, scar tissue, wrinkles and varicose veins.

I have seen MSM be of value in the treatment of emphysema, joint pain, allergies and chemical sensitivities. It has also been reported to be effective in certain stomach and digestive tract conditions, circulation disorders and the control of parasites. Several months ago I saw a patient who was confined to a wheelchair. Just recently, she walked into my office with the partial aid of a walker. She thanked me profusely for giving her MSM, which, she was sure, helped her walk again.

I spend a considerable amount of time walking in the deserts and mountains, with exposure to poisonous snakes and scorpions. I find it comforting to know that MSM and Microhydrin are two substances that counter the effects of snakebites, fleabites, spider-bites and bee stings. Microhydrin works in much the same way as MSM; however, it is a different antioxidant and much more potent. It can relieve stiff sore muscles, increase your energy, and decrease your sensitivity to sunlight. It is very useful in helping one's allergies. It also has been found to inhibit cardiovascular disease, stimulate the adrenal glands and eliminate some bacterial and viral infections. Anyone exposed to any form of pollution, or whose immune system is compromised for any reason, would benefit from using Microhydrin.

NSC-24 is a very powerful immune defense formula extracted from yeast cell walls. It helps to prevent repeated infections and is also useful in treating acute parasite, viral and yeast infections. NSC-24 has been successful in fighting some cancers, as well as in reducing the effects of aging, allergies and chronic fatigue syndrome. Several months ago a patient with persistent pneumonia was not responding well to very powerful antibiotics. He was treated with NSC-24 and the pneumonia was resolved. Another patient with a strep throat did not test well with kinesiology for *any* antibiotic. This was my first patient with strep who was unresponsive to any antibiotic. I fear this is the beginning of a trend. Thankfully, the patient tested well for NSC-24. Another patient with a sinus infection who was treated for over six weeks with antibiotics was not responding and was scheduled for sinus surgery, which the patient feared. She also did not test well for any antibiotic but did for NSC-24. She was very grateful when seven days later her symptoms were gone and her x-ray was back to normal.

MGN-3 was first brought to my attention by Dr. David Williams in his newsletter "Alternatives" (Volume 7, #15), September 1998. He described how Dr. Ghoneum did research to show that MGN-3 is a very powerful immune system booster. It is produced from the outer shell of rice bran and the extracts from three different mushrooms. It has been shown to increase the activity of our white blood cells, specifically our natural killer cells. It also increases our interferon level, which is the formation of tumor necrosis factor proteins. It has been found beneficial in treating infections and cancer. It is in cancer that I have found it to be very helpful; especially in prostate cancer. It has been reported to be effective also in ovarian and breast cancer. One patient with multiple myeloma also experienced complete remissions!

Transfer Factor and Transfer Factor Plus are recent immune boosters, comprised mainly of colostrum. In the past two weeks I have had two patients with bacterial infections that did not test with kinesiology for any antibiotic or nutritional supplement other than Transfer Factor Plus. I was sure happy that I had something to offer them to combat their infection. I have used it myself on three occasions to treat staph infections with prompt, excellent results.

Herbs

There is an increasing use of herbal products by American consumers. A 1997 survey revealed that thirty-two percent of American adults spent an average of fifty-four dollars per year on herbal remedies. Herbs in general are quite safe but can cause some adverse side effects, i.e., individual sensitivity, toxic reaction and occasionally negative interactions with prescription drugs. Although confirmed reports of harmful effects are rare (the World Health Organization has reported only 5,000 cases of suspected adverse reactions to herbal medicines), caution is needed with these products. Again, I stress the importance of kinesiology.

It is important to remember that herbal extracts are stronger than tinctures. Generally, small frequent doses are better tolerated than large, infrequent doses. A solid extract is more concentrated, stable and economical than a fluid extract. Make certain that you take a fresh, standardized whole herb preparation and follow the directions regarding the proper dose.

Cayenne Pepper
Cayenne pepper is an herb that should be in every home. It is great for your circulation. If you suspect that a person is having a heart attack, give them a heaping teaspoon of cayenne pepper in a glass of water while you wait for the ambulance. It could mean the difference between life and death. It can also slow both internal and external bleeding.

Lobelia
Another favorite herb is Lobelia. It has been effective in the relief of respiratory illnesses.

Echinacea
Echinacea comes from a daisy and enhances the lymphatic system. It is also an immune system stimulator that can increase the white blood cells in your body to help fight infection. Preliminary test results show an increase in interferon hormone levels as well.

Elderberry
Elderberry (Sambucus Nigra) has been successful in the treatment of viral infections—especially those involving the throat—when used within the first two to three days of the onset of the illness.

Goldenseal
Goldenseal (Hydricus Candedensis) is another good herb for infections primarily of the mucosa but not during pregnancy. It is more anti-bacterial than Elderberry.

Pao d'Arco
Pao d'Arco (Tabebuia Rosea) is a tree bark extract often used as a tea. It is very good for systemic infections, candida and other fungus infections. Pao d'Arco has also been effective against certain types of cancer.

Yarrow

Yarrow (Acheillea Milleflovim) can be used as a urinary antiseptic as well as to reduce some fevers.

St. John's Wort

St. John's Wort (Hypericum). Recently, considerable attention has been created in the medical and lay press regarding the use of St. John's Wort as a treatment for depression. It is also an antiviral medication found to be helpful in some cases of HIV. Like Elderberry, it should be used in the early stages of an infection for best results.

Boneset

Boneset (Eupatorium) has been found effective in treating influenza, while decreasing aches, pains and fever.

Two others, *Myrrh* and *Hyssop,* are both useful as anti-microbial and antiviral agents.

Saw Palmetto

Saw Palmetto has been proven in a random "double" blind study to be effective in treating benign prostatic enlargement.

Feverfew

Feverfew is used for long-term migraine headache management. Both the severity *and* frequency of migraine headaches can be addressed.

Ginseng

Ginseng has been used for over 2,500 years. Atherosclerosis, hypertension, male infertility, erectile dysfunction and diabetes have been successfully treated with this popular herb. Ginseng has also been effective in lowering the risk of some cancers.

Astragalus

Astragalus is very effective in boosting the immune system, increasing energy and maximizing the effects of ginseng.

Valerian Root

Valerian Root is widely used for insomnia and anxiety.

Kava Kava

Kava Kava is also excellent for reducing anxiety and enhancing relaxation. It comes from the South Pacific and has proven itself when compared to prescription drugs such as Serax. It should not be used during pregnancy or with other prescription tranquilizers or antidepressants, or even with St. John's Wort.

Ginger

Ginger was used as early as 4,000 B.C. It can reduce the effects of motion sickness and improve digestion. It is an anti-inflammatory and a pain reliever. It also reduces cholesterol levels.

Olive Leaf

The bible contains many references to olive leaf. Now it has been found to be of tremendous value in treating almost all infections—bacterial, viral, yeast, and so forth. It has also been found to be beneficial for diabetes and hypertension and has been shown to cure psoriasis. It is truly a wonderful medicinal herb.

Collosonia Root

This herb is wonderful for treating hemorrhoids. I have prescribed this for over twenty years with over ninety-percent reduction in the need for hemorrhoidectomy.

Larrea Tridentata (Chaparral)

A desert bush has been found to be very effective against the many viruses in the Herpes family. One of which is Cytomegalourus which has been incriminated in the development of heart disease and high blood pressure. It may also be useful in post-operation heart surgery cases. A safe natural product containing Larrea is available as Larreastat. To obtain this as well as other products discussed in this chapter, refer to the last page of this chapter.

Arguna

Terminalea arguna tree is found in India. Bark preparations have been used to treat heart conditions for over 2,000 years. The bark not only lowers total cholesterol but also LDL, which is the harmful cholesterol. It has been found to relieve angina and inhibit atherosclerosis. Another interesting property is its ability to have significant antibacterial activity and to have cancer-fighting properties. It is available under the name Arguna-Cardiac Tonic.

Lyprinol (New Zealand green-lipped mussel)
This has been found very useful in reducing pain and stiffness (inflammation) in arthritic conditions. Even though it is excellent for pain, it will not rebuild damaged cartilage, so it should be used in conjunction with glucosamine and chrondroitin.

Sea Cucumber
This contains natural chrondroitin and glucosamine. A brand called Flexanol contains this plus MSM, ginger root, borageoil, vitamins C & E and boswellian serrata to repair joint damage and decrease pain.

Benefin
A shark cartilage product that not only helps arthritis symptoms but also is a natural cancer therapy.

Nexrutin
Phellodendron Amurense—has been used in Chinese medicine for over 1,000 years to treat pain and arthritis symptoms. It has been shown in clinical study to be on the average of seventy percent effective for pain relief within seven days in patients with arthritis and fibromyalgia.

Huperzine A
Chinese club moss—huperziaserrata. Found useful in the treatment and prevention of brain aging such as Alzheimer's disease and age-related cognitive decline.

Remiary 1 (galantamine)
Approved by the FDA in March 2001 for use in Alzheimer's disease, it is an extract from the snowdrop, daffodil, spider lily and other plants. Parkinson disease and multiple sclerosis patients may also benefit from its use.

Rhododendron Caucasicum (snow rose)
Grows at ten to thirty thousand feet in the Caucasus Mountains in the Republic of Georgia (previously in the Soviet Union). Its people are renowned for their longevity, with many living in excess of one-hundred years. It has been found to be beneficial for a multitude of medical problems such as arthritis, heart disease, hypertension, depression, psychoses and concentration problems.

Lycopene
Strong antioxidant found in tomatoes, pink gradefruit, watermelon and apricots. It is thought to decrease the risk of cancer, especially in the prostate, stomach and lung.

Alpha-lipoic acid (sulfur containing fatty acid)
Helps to convert blood sugar into energy and is an antioxidant. Used in treatment of diabetes, cataracts, Parkinson's disease and Alzheimer's disease.

Modified citrus pectin
First nontoxic therapy that naturally and specifically interferes with cancer metastasis. Don't confuse MCP with natural citrus pectin, the kind that is common in health food stores.

Silymarin
Silymarin from milk thistle and artichokes has been used for over 2,000 years to treat liver problems. I have found it to be very useful in my practice. In the past ten years it has been found to be very effective for colon and skin cancer, and perhaps even breast cancer.

Phytochemicals
They give plants their color, smell and flavor. These natural substances are very important to our health and immune systems. Some of the more important sources of phytochemicals are:

Broccoli
Three-day-old broccoli sprouts may decrease the size and amount of breast tumors due to a chemical called silforaphene. Also found in cabbage, kale and cauliflower. A very well-known medical friend of mine told me before he died that he believed that broccoli's main therapeutic property was organic arsenic.

Green Tea
Green tea contains polyphenols that help to decrease LDL, the harmful cholesterol. Polyphenols also block nitrosamines that are found in fish and meat due to processing and cooking. They are powerful antioxidants that destroy free radicals and other toxins as well as inhibit the clotting factor called thromboxane A2, for which aspirin is recommended.

Turmeric

A spice that has been used for years in Greek and Chinese medicine for liver disorders, menstrual disorders, inflammation, eczema and hemorrhage.

Phytochemical Supplements

Phytochemical supplements are available from several different sources. Some of the best products contain synergistic mixtures of several of those discussed above.

AHCC

AHCC is an activated hexose correlate compound. Only recently has this been available in the United States. It is an extract of several different medical mushrooms and has been used with very good results in Japan for people with cancer and AIDS and other very serious illnesses. It is also an excellent promoter of good health by strengthening immune systems. It is one of the world's safeest and most powerful immune stimulators. Available as ImmPower.

As I try to emphasize throughout this book, it is very important to shift our focus from disease-specific interventions to the fundamental underlying causes of health and disease. To improve our immune systems—not only to prevent but to treat the many medical problems that we face in the world today—must be our goal. Before treating yourself with various herbal combinations, you should seek all treatment options and consult with medical personnel who can help you make a wise decision if they are informed about alternative medicine.

Biotics Research, DSD
11001 N. 24th Ave., Suite 603
Phoenix, Arizona 85029
1-800-232-3183

These can be ordered if you are under the care of a physician. Some of the ones I use most frequently are:

ADP

ADP is an oregano extract excellent for systemic yeast infections and some parasitic infections.

ADHS

ADHS is helpful for acute adrenal insufficiency and fatigue.

Cytozyme AD
Cytozyme AD is used for chronic adrenal insufficiency.

BetaPlus & Beta TCP
BetaPlus & Beta TCP are both used for liver and gall bladder problems.

Biocardiozyme Forte
Biocardiozyme Forte strengthens the heart muscle.

Bioglycozyme Forte and Glucobalance
Bioglycozyme Forte and Glucobalance are multivitamins for diabetes.

Crzyme & Vzyme
Crzyme & vzyme are two minerals important in the treatment of diabetes.

E-mulsion 200
E-mulsion 200 is a very useful form of vitamin E.

Equifem
Equifem is a multiple vitamin for post-menstrual women.

Folic acid & Bio 6
Folic acid & Bio 6 are helpful in the prevention of heart disease.

Bio B 100
Bio B 100 is a natural form of multiple B vitamins.

Osteo B Plus
Osteo B Plus is helpful for osteoporosis.

Iron-copper Free Multi Plus
Iron-copper Free Multi Plus is a multiple vitamin designed for persons living in areas that have high levels of iron and copper deposits. Too much iron in our system definitely diminishes our immune system, so we must avoid its over-use.

Porphrazyme
Porphrazyme is my personal favorite oral chelator to treat heavy metal toxicity and I find great usefor it in treating coronary artery disease. I usually use it prior to I.V. chelation with EDTA.

Flax Seed oil caps

Flax Seed oil in a caps format is one of my top recommendations for almost everyone from ADD children to all women. Also a big help to everyone in improving their circulation problems.

Biotics Research also has many other products that help with hormonal, vitamin and mineral deficiencies. I have found their brand of amino acids and neonatal glandulars to be the best available.

It is always wise to remember that in nutrition, as in most instances, moderation is the preferred choice; too little is not good and too much is definitely to be avoided.

Through the years I have obtained the information I have presented here from many, many different sources. I wish to thank them all—books, newsletters, nutritional articles, and so forth. I have discussed primarily those which I have used or tested. For up to date specialized information on products and sources of purchase, I suggest your becoming a member of the Health Science Institute, Members Services Department, 819 North Charles St., Baltimore, Maryland 21201, Telephone: (508) 368-7494, Fax: (410) 230-1273. Their publications discuss many more alternative nutritional products that may well be of benefit to you or your loved ones. I have not discussed them here because I have not yet had the opportunity to test and/or use them.

Consider for a moment some common mistakes made by energetic people trying to improve their health. The most frequently made error of enthusiasm is the purchase of calcium in the form of oyster shell or calcium carbonate. Less than ten percent of calcium carbonate is absorbed, yet it is the most widely recommended calcium salt. Calcium carbonate performs well as an antacid. However, we need the stomach acid to help digest and absorb the calcium. Overuse of calcium carbonate is a self-defeating process. If you're using calcium carbonate you might as well save your time and just dump it directly into the toilet. If you want to use it as an antacid, that's perfectly fine, but don't rely upon it as a good source of calcium.

One of the better readily available calcium salts is calcium citrate. Compared to calcium carbonate it is much more highly absorbed. There are many different kinds of calcium salts with much better absorption rates than calcium carbonate, including calcium oratate, calcium aspartame, calcium lactate and calcium gluconate. Of these, the best one is calcium oratate. Unfortunately this product is not currently available in the United States except in a form that is not as effective as the source from Germany.

Probably the second most common mistake is the purchase of vitamin E, dl-alpha, the synthetic form of vitamin E. In my opinion the synthetic form of vitamin E produces numerous side effects detrimental to the immune system. I have been using high doses of vitamin E in the majority of my patients since 1970 and have not yet seen any side effects from the vitamin E, providing it is d Alpha.

Last year a patient came into the office with a large trash bag full of supplements she was currently taking. I didn't count each one, but the bag was so heavy she had trouble lifting it. It is my guess that she had over one-hundred different supplements. She told me she was taking most of them on a daily basis. She had been working at a health food store in Phoenix and was convinced that all of them were good for something and therefore good for her. I tested each one with kinesiology and only about ten percent agreed with her. She became quite agitated when I suggested she cut down on the number of supplements. She expressed concern about not being able to get by without them. I said it should be the other way around. "How can you take so many supplements that don't agree with you? What about the inevitable side effects?" She left the office and I haven't seen her since.

Minerals

Mineral supplementation is even more critical to good health than vitamin supplementation. Our bodies are lacking in minerals largely due to the mineral deficiency of our soils. If the grains and plants don't get fed, then neither do you. Minerals are the basic foundation of our structure. Some vitamins can be produced through photosynthesis, but not minerals. According to Senate Document 264; our soil has been "officially" deficient in minerals since 1936. The 1992 Earth Summit concluded that the mineral content in our soils has not improved. The United States has, on average, the poorest farming soil in the world! This is probably one of the reasons that we have more health problems than the Europeans even though we spend twice as much on health care.

The World Health Organization rated the United States eighteenth in the world for longevity, nineteenth for degenerative diseases and twenty-third for infant survival! It is interesting to compare the foods our animals eat to our own. Dog food has over forty minerals added, rabbit food over twenty-five and baby food only eleven.

There are numerous mineral compositions called "salts." For example, we have calcium carbonate and calcium citrate. When reading the amount of calcium in a tablet, for example, you have to know the amount of elemental calcium and not be confused by the salt content. The compound (salt) the mineral is attached to makes a difference in its effectiveness and absorption. Calcium, such as dolomite, is a ground-up rock deposit with an absorption rate of less than five percent. Many years ago a chemical process known as chelating was developed to coat the mineral with an amino acid and increase the absorption level to forty percent.

There are other forms of mineral salts with even better absorption rates, such as the oratates. All of these factors have to be taken into consideration when selecting or prescribing a mineral supplement. As we have mentioned earlier, calcium carbonate is good as an antacid but not good as a calcium supplement. It is not well absorbed and, when absorbed, is often deposited in vessels and soft tissue where obviously it is not wanted. One of the reasons it is not good as a calcium supplement is that it decreases the stomach acid needed for absorption of calcium. To make it even more complicated, there are two forms of carbonate, seven citrates, five gluconates and fourteen lactates.

Some of the more common minerals and the areas they affect are:

Area or Condition	Mineral
Adrenal	Chloride, Sodium
Blood	Iron, Copper, Calcium, Molybdenum*
Bone, joints	Calcium, Magnesium, Potassium, Phosphorus, Boron, Manganese, Zinc, Copper
Diabetes	Chromium, Vanadium, Selenium*, Magnesium, Copper, Manganese, Zinc, Potassium, Calcium
Eyes	Copper, Zinc
Heart	Calcium, Copper, Chromium, Magnesium, Manganese, Potassium, Selenium*, Vanadium, Zinc
Immune System	Copper, Manganese, Zinc, Selenium*, Magnesium
Infertility	Zinc, Magnesium
Muscles-Skeletal	Sodium, Calcium, Magnesium, Potassium, Selenium*, Phosphorus, Manganese
Prostate	Magnesium, Zinc, Selenium*
Thyroid	Iodine, Magnesium, Copper, Manganese, Selenium*, Rubidium*

* Trace Mineral

Don't underestimate the importance of trace minerals. These are minerals your body needs in very small amounts. Even though only small quantities are required, deficiencies can cause acute health problems.

In addition to chromium, selenium and vanadium, other trace minerals such as germanium, rubidium, lithium, silver, molybdenum and cobalt have been used successfully to treat a wide variety of symptoms. There are many more trace minerals, but the aforementioned have proven to be most beneficial.

In my experience one of the best-absorbed mineral salts is the oratates made in Germany. Previously we were able to obtain them here in the United States. There is a company here that makes oratates but they are not the same as the oratates from Germany and do not work as well, so I very rarely use them now. Oratates are the mineral salts of vitamin B_{13} and are one of the most effective salts available for absorption and therapeutic effect. They are produced when orotic acid combines with a mineral and is a key molecule in the formation of the nucleic acids DNA and RNA. The absorption rate of the oratates is sixty to eighty percent compared to the phosphates, carbonates and oxides that have an absorption rate of only one to nine percent. Some of the oratates and the conditions they have helped are as follows:

Mineral Salt	Conditions
Calcium oratate	multiple sclerosis, asthma, hepatitis and cirrhosis, arthritis, cardiovascular functioning
Magnesium oratate Note: *should not be taken at the same time as Calcium Oratate*	psoriasis, heart function, angina, atherosclerosis, kidney stones, insomnia, digestive problems
Potassium oratate	heart function, myocarditis, angina, arrythymias
Lithium oratate	migraine, depression, alcoholism, epilepsy— when taken with calcium oratate a great improvement in liver function has been reported
Zinc oratate	Works on both benign and malignant tumors to shrink them—also effective against long-lasting infections and diabetes

Several cases come to mind that I treated twenty years ago when these supplements were available.

- My good friend, a pharmacist, had a hunting dog who was so crippled with arthritis that he was unable to hunt, and my friend was very sad and was thinking of perhaps having to put his dog to sleep. After starting the dog on calcium oratate, the arthritis disappeared and the dog was able to hunt for several more years. My friend has been forever grateful.

- The sister of my best friend in Ishpeming had brain cancer and had two operations for it. The neurosurgeon was unable to remove all the tumor and she was given six months to live. We started her on zinc oratate and she improved. She was still living three years later when I left there!

- An elderly gentleman with severe Alzheimer's was a patient in a nursing home I attended. He had a squamous cell carcinoma the size of a large orange on the left side of his face. Because of his condition, the family refused surgery or radiation. I placed him on zinc oratate and one year later to the day, the cancer was completely gone.

- I have had numerous other cases, particularly cardiovascular that cleared on calcium, potassium and magnesium oratate.

Recently I have become acquainted with Mr. Fred Eichorn. He had to drop out of medical school because of a pancreatic cancer. He treated himself with a specific nutritional supplement he created, and he was cured. Since then he has treated many cancer victims with amazing results. So far almost all types of cancers have responded. He has also found it very beneficial in other non-cancer conditions such as diabetes, hepatitis C and many other conditions.

Amino Acids

The discussion of amino acids can be very complicated and prolonged. Entire textbooks have been written on the subject. In most cases amino acids can be used in place of allopathic medication without concern for side effects. The following is a review of some of the more common amino acids and their therapeutic benefits.

L-Arginine
The dosage range is between 500 and 3,000 milligrams twice a day. L-Arginine has been beneficial in reducing the size of cancerous tumors. It has been used to treat

some forms of hair loss, especially if the hair is dry and breaking. Burn patients and patients with infections experience increases in the immune system function with improved wound healing. Other uses include the control of fatty livers, lowering cholesterol, lowering blood pressure and the treatment of Raynaud's Disease and impotency. When used with vitamin B-5 and Choline, L-Arginine increases the release of human growth hormone, a potent deterrent to the effects of aging. I recommend that L-Arginine be taken on an empty stomach.

L-Carnitine

The normal dosage for L-Carnitine is 600 milligrams three times a day. I have used it with good results in patients with high triglyceride levels. L-Carnitine can be used in place of Lopid and other cholesterol medications. It is also a vasodilator, which is especially useful in diabetic cases. Like L-Arginine, L-Carnitine will lower blood pressure. It's very beneficial for anyone on kidney dialysis and can be useful in cases of cirrhosis. In high doses, L-Carnitine can promote muscle energy; however, the effects may not be seen for two to four weeks.

L-Cysteine

This is one of my favorite amino acids for alternative therapy. L-Cysteine is extremely beneficial to patients with asthma and is essential to any detoxification process. Patients attempting to increase their HDL cholesterol levels and decrease their triglycerides can benefit from L-Cysteine. It is an excellent detoxifier in cases of diabetic kidney failure and liver disease. It can also eliminate lead, cobalt, molybdenum and cadmium from the body. L-Cysteine has been effective in treating allergic reactions, smoker's cough and some cases of psoriasis and rheumatoid arthritis. The daily intake should not exceed 4,000 milligrams.

L-Lysine

I have had my best success with this amino acid treating virus infections. In most patients, a dosage of 1,000 milligrams four times a day is adequate.

L-Phenylalanine

L-Phenylaline is used primarily for pain reduction and the alleviation of depression. It exerts a lot of its influence by degrading into Tyrosine. For pain reduction, the dl form is better. I have also found it useful in some cases of attention deficit disorder. People using this amino acid should avoid caffeine, as it tends to decrease the serum levels. The usual dosage is one-and-one-half to three grams twice a day.

Methinione

Methinione can be used for a number of conditions, including drug detoxification, allergies, depression, heavy metal toxicity and elevated cholesterol levels. It has been reported to be somewhat effective against Parkinson's disease, although the effects are unpredictable. One of its major attributes is to protect the body against radiation.

L-Histadine

L-Histadine has been helpful in the treatment of rheumatoid arthritis, schizophrenia, and hyperactivity. The average dosage is one-half to one gram three times a day. Serum levels can be measured. Low levels may contribute to cataract formation. L-Histadine is a good vasodilator.

L-Tyrosine

I have had good success in treating depression with this amino acid. It is often more effective than Prozac, Zoloft and some of the other more common antidepressants. In small doses, L-Tyrosine increases appetite and in large doses it decreases appetite. This amino acid also stimulates the libido and increases the sex drive. Used over a period of time L-Tyrosine increases one's endurance. The normal dosage is 1 to 3 grams a day.

L-Tryptophane

L-Trytophane is an excellent alternative for reducing stress and insomnia. It was taken off the market several years ago; however, it can now be purchased by prescription.

L-Taurine

L-Taurine has been found effective in cases of edema, epilepsy, photophobia, macular degeneration, depression, obesity and occasionally hypertension. It improves gall bladder function by increasing bile flow and cutting down on bile stasis. Doses of approximately 3,000 milligrams have been used to successfully treat congestive heart failure. 500 to 1,000 milligrams is the standard dose. It can increase sperm motility, help mitral valve prolapse, and improve some cases of cardiomyopathy.

GABA (Gamma-amino-buteric-acid)

This useful amino acid has been used in the treatment of Parkinson's disease. It helps decrease appetite and balance blood sugar levels, hence it is very useful to both diabetics and hypoglycemics. GABA is a great nutritional supplement for anxiety, depression and epilepsy. It metabolizes into L-Glutamine. It will also help lower blood pressure. The usual dosage is two to three grams per day in undivided doses.

L-Glutamine

This amino acid has been used successfully in cases of infertility and depression. It can also help with anorexia and headaches. I use L-Glutamine extensively for my patients withdrawing from alcohol. To be effective, twenty to thirty of the 500-milligram capsules a day are required. In this instance natural B vitamins, zinc, magnesium and a good multivitamin should be added to the treatment regimen. L-Glutamine can increase tumor growth, so it must be avoided by anyone with cancer.

These are just a few of the amino acids that can be used to help counter many disease processes and oftentimes replace allopathic medication. Amino acids can be used as a good example of the differences between brands and quality. There are five different nutritional grades of amino acids, from the worst to the best. Obviously, if you take an inferior amino acid it might not work at all or just a little. If you take an amino acid and don't get the expected results, it could be that it was of poor quality or possibly it was because you did not have enough stomach acid to properly digest and assimilate it. There are many factors to consider.

You can take the proper nutrition, but if your digestive system is not working properly to digest and assimilate the nutrition, it will seem as if the nutritional products are not working. Some claim that most illness starts in a poorly functioning digestive system. Based on my experience, I would agree that many of our current illnesses start or are worsened by a gastrointestinal tract that is performing less than optimally because of unwise food selection, chemicals, antibiotics, insufficient water and infection.

Food Allergies

Hippocrates said, "Thy food shall be thy remedy." I agree, however, food is also often thy illness. Each day I encounter the common, under-diagnosed condition of food allergy. The symptoms are usually overlooked by the attending physician or are attributed to another illness. In this regard I recommend that you read *Allergies—Disease in Disguise,* by Carolee Kock, D.C., N.D.

Dr. James Brenemen, a general practitioner from Galesburg, Michigan, introduced me to the concept of food allergy during my internship at Borgess

Hospital. Since 1961 I have been totally convinced that food allergy is a major, undetected problem. Allergies to food can cause skin rashes, constipation, diarrhea, migraine and common headaches, arthritis, fatigue, depression, bed-wetting, hoarseness, sneezing, wheezing, anaphylactic shock, eczema, hyperactivity, asthma, hives, cramping, gas and nausea and many other symptoms. I specifically evaluate my patients for food allergies. I have had patients undergo skin tests and RAST (blood) tests; however, they are expensive and often misleading. Therefore, I rarely use them unless the patient requests them. In the past, I relied on the Elimination Diet pioneered by Dr. Breneman. With the Elimination Diet, the patient diets for 15 days and gradually adds back one "pure" food and watches for symptoms.

Following is the original Elimination Diet developed by Dr. Breneman. It is still a valuable tool for those who do not have access to, or who do not believe in, kinesiology. It may help you determine the cause of your symptoms.

Elimination Diet—Foods You May Eat

Category	Food
Condiments	Salts, sugar
Beverage	Tea (only sugar may be added)
Bread	Rice wafers
Cereal	Rice; white, brown wild, puffed, flour
Fruits	All must be thoroughly cooked; nothing added by sugar Apricots, cherries: dried, fresh, frozen home and commercially canned Peaches: canned, if only sugar added Cranberries and Prunes
Fats	Lamb fat drippings, Olive oil
Fruit Juice	Apricot Cranberry: homemade and commercially canned if only sugar added Prune: only sugar added
Meat	Lamb
Miscellaneous	Ripe olives, Vanilla extract (pure) Baking soda, Tapioca (pure) Salt, Cream of Tartar Gelatin (pure and Citric Acid [purchased from a drug store] non-flavored)
Sweets	Sugars (white or brown) Sugar syrups (homemade) Sugar and water candies (pure, homemade) Jams and preserves (homemade from allowed fruits and sugars)
Vegetables	All must be thoroughly cooked. Seasoned only with salt and allowed fats. Beets: fresh, frozen, home and commercially canned if only salt added Beet greens: fresh Spinach: fresh, frozen, home and commercially canned if only salt and sugar added.

Sample Menu

Breakfast	Lunch	Dinner
Cream of rice or Rice Krispies	Lamb Chops (broil)	Roast Lamb
Rice Wafers	Sweet Potatoes	Rice
Stewed Prunes	Beets or Beet Greens	Spinach with vinegar
Apricot or Prune Juice	Ripe Olives	Apricot salad
Tea	Rice wafers	Rice wafers
	Canned peaches	Canned Cherries
	Tea	Tea

After following the above elimination diet for 15+ days, if you don't improve, you may be allergic to rice or one of the other foods on the diet. If you feel better, add back one "pure" food each two days, such as milk, tomato or wheat and not a mixture of new foods. Add the new food for breakfast in a large amount. If there is no reaction, or a questionable reaction, add again for lunch and dinner. If there is no adverse reaction, add larger quantities the second day. At this point, if there is no adverse effect, the food can be added to your diet. The following steps outline the process of adding foods back into your diet.

Steps—Starting on the 15th Day:

1. Add back milk, wheat, eggs, chicken, tomatoes, corn, beef, and so on.

2. Add back one pure food at a time–usually daily if feeling well. Do not try a new food if you're not feeling well.

3. Add back food in large quantity and add back at breakfast always and note whether there is no reaction, a questionable or a positive reaction.

4. If food is OK—add to basic diet.

5. If a positive reaction develops:

    a. Stop food

    b. List symptoms

    c. Retry in 2 weeks

6. If symptoms persist: also remove food from day before reaction started (delayed reaction) Usually each allergic food will produce different symptoms, i.e., one might cause a rash, another might produce asthma symptoms, while yet another may give you gastrointestinal problems. Many patients find this process too difficult. I now utilize the applied kinesiology techniques fostered by Dr. George Goodhart to diagnose food allergies.

Food Allergy Record Keeping

Directions:
As you add back foods to your diet, you'll want to record your body's reaction. Use the blank chart on the next page as a guide. Either photocopy the chart or follow the layout to create your own.

Use the first column to record the food you're adding back to your diet and add a check mark in column two to indicate whether you experience a reaction.

The sample chart on this page includes a number of possible symptoms that are common among people who have food allergies.

Sample

Food	Reaction	Symptoms
	____ No Reaction ____ (?) Reaction ____ Positive Reaction	Rash Stomach Upset Diarrhea Headache Fatigue Irritability Depression Arthritic symptoms Pain Swelling Painful urination

Food Allergy Chart

Food	Reaction	Symptoms
	_____ No Reaction _____ (?) Reaction _____ Positive Reaction	
	_____ No Reaction _____ (?) Reaction _____ Positive Reaction	
	_____ No Reaction _____ (?) Reaction _____ Positive Reaction	
	_____ No Reaction _____ (?) Reaction _____ Positive Reaction	
	_____ No Reaction _____ (?) Reaction _____ Positive Reaction	
	_____ No Reaction _____ (?) Reaction _____ Positive Reaction	

Small amounts of molybdenum (150 to 450 milligrams) will decrease food sensitivity. Mo-Zyme and Allerplex can also be helpful. My primary treatment of food allergies focuses on avoidance. This can be especially difficult with what I call "hidden foods." These are widely represented on the grocer's shelves. The following list of common foods can help you identify and avoid "hidden foods" in other products. Carefully read labels and don't hesitate to make inquiries if you have any doubt as to a food's contents.

Egg

Baking powders	Hamburger Mix	Pancake Flour
Bavarian Cream	Hollandaise Sauce	Puddings
Breaded Foods	Ice Cream	Salad Dressings
Breads	Icings	Sauces
Cake Flours	Macaroni	Sausages
Cakes	Macaroons	Sherbets
French Toast	Marshmallows	Soufflés
Fritters	Mayonnaise	Tartar Sauce
Frostings	Meat Loaf	Waffles
Frying Batters Glazed	Meat Molds	Wines
Rolls	Meringues	
Griddle Cakes	Noodles	

Yeast

Barbecue Sauce	Fruit Juices	Salad Dressing
Beer	Gin	Soy Sauce
Brandy	Malted Milk	Tomato Sauce
Breads	Mayonnaise	Truffles
Buttermilk	Mince Pie	Vinegar
Cakes	Olives	Vodka
Cereals	Pastries	Vitamins
Cheeses	Buns, and so forth	Whiskey
Condiments	Pickles	Wine
Cookies	Pretzels	Yogurt
Crackers	Rolls	
Enriched Flours	Rum	

Wheat

Beer	Bread	Ice Cream
Biscuits	Crackers	Liverwurst
Bologna	Cocomalt	Lunch Ham
Bouillon Cubes	Doughnuts	Macaroni
Cakes	Dumplings	Matzos
Cereals	Flour-rolled Meats	
Cookies	Flour	
Cooked Meat Dishes	Gluten	
Chocolate	Bread	
Candy	Gravies	
Corn	Griddle Cakes	

Corn

Aspirin	Distilled Vinegar	Margarine
Baking Powder	Doughnuts	Pancake Mix
Beer, Ale	Fat-Frying Mix	Pie Crusts
Biscuits	Fritos	Popcorn
Bleached Flour Breads	Frozen Fruits	Powdered Sugar
Pastries	Frozen Vegetables	Preserves
Cakes, Cookies	Frying Batters	Puddings, Custards
Candies	Glucose Products	Salad Dressing
Carbonated Bevs	Graham Crackers	Soups (creamed)
Catsup	Gravies	Starch
Chewing Gum	Grits	Toothpaste
Cough Syrup	Ice Cream, Sherbet	Tortillas
Cream Pies	Instant Teas	Vitamins
Cured Hams	Jams	Whiskey
Dates (Confections)	Jellies	

Soybeans

Baby Foods	Ice Cream	Salad Dressings
Biscuits	Lecithin	Soups
Breads	Lunch Meats	Soy Flour
Butter Substitute	Margarine	Soy Noodles
Cake	Milk Substitute	Tempura
Caramel	Nut Candies	Tofu
Cereals	Oils	
Crackers	Oriental Sauces	
Crisco Spray	Pastries	
Hard Candies	Pork Link Sausages	

Milk

Au Gratin Foods	Custards	Salad Dressings
Bavarian Cream	Doughnuts	Scalloped Dishes
Biscuits	Flour Mixes	Sherbets
Breads	Fritters	Soda Crackers
Buttermilk	Gravies	Soufflés
Cakes	Ice Cream	Soups
Cookies	Mashed Potatoes	Spumoni
Candies	Omelettes	Waffles
Cheeses	Ovaltine	Whey Yogurt
Chowders	Ovamalt	
Cocoa Drinks	Pancakes	
Creamed Foods	Pie Crusts	
Curds	Rarebits	

If you can avoid a certain food for several months, your sensitivity to it may decrease to the point where you can eat small amounts every fourth or fifth day.

I have had hundreds of success stories treating patients for food allergy, and I could write a book about this subject with some very interesting and happy outcomes. However, my first case still is very clear in my mind and is a good example to relate. I mentioned the case briefly in a previous chapter.

I was a senior at the University of Michigan on a private medical staff of one of the most respected doctors at the University. I was very privileged to have been chosen to be on his staff. He had a patient—a forty-five-year-old lady—whose problem was chronic diarrhea. She was an inpatient for over three weeks and was given every test available and tried numerous medications all to no avail. She left the hospital unimproved and somewhat despondent.

Several months later after graduation, I interned at Borgess Hospital in Kalamazoo and there met Dr. Brenaman from Galesberg. He taught me about food allergies, and I thought of the lady with the chronic diarrhea. I called her and had her make an appointment with Dr. Brenaman. He hospitalized her briefly to speed up her detoxification with intravenous fluids and ACTH. After identifying her food allergies and eliminating them, her diarrhea cleared up!

So in 1960 at a most prestigious Medical University, food allergy as a problem was not entertained.

NAET is a technique that has been found to be very valuable for correcting allergies of all kinds. If you have allergies that need correction, be sure to search and find a practitioner that specializes in NAET therapy (allergy elimination technique). N stands for the woman's name that devised the therapy; A for Allergy, E for Elimination and T for Technique. With this technique you can often get rid of your allergies for *life*!

As a person with many allergies, I have been treated with NAET and have benefited greatly. I am truly pleased. I have referred dozens of my patients for this treatment with very good results.

NAET can not only eliminate food allergies but also pollen, grass, environmental allergies, and so forth. It is a life saver for the chemical-sensitive and multi-allergy sufferers. So if this pertains to you, find the best NAET practitioner in your area and start to feel better. There is also a good possibility that even patients with fibromyalgia will benefit from this technique! It is noninvasive, and uses no needles, and so on Again, the use of kinesiology is an important diagnostic application in its use.

Hypothyroidism

Sub-clinical hypothyroidism is a medical problem that many physicians don't believe exists, much less requires treatment. The majority of medical doctors will treat hypothyroid symptoms *only* if the blood test reflects hypothyroidism. The fact that many patients have multiple symptoms with subclinical hypothyroidism does not impress these physicians. Since many of these symptoms can be associated with other conditions including food allergies, they are usually ignored.

Since I have been in practice, many thyroid tests have come and gone beginning with the Basal Metabolic Rate (BMR). There was also the Protein Bound Iodine (PBI) and the Achilles reflex test, and so on. Now we have tests to measure the T3 thyroid fraction in addition to the T4 fraction. Presently the most sensitive test is the TSH (thyroid stimulating hormone). I feel that thyroid treatment is a good example of how a physician should practice medicine. He should take a very thorough history, listen to the patient, do a complete exam (preferably along with kinesiology) and then treat the patient and not the blood test.

In Dr. Broda Barns' book on hypothyroidism it was noted that a low basal morning temperature (ninety-six to ninety-seven degrees under the arm) was one sign of low thyroid. This I agree with, but I believe it can also be a sign of low pituitary. There is much controversy over treating subclinical hypothyroidism, but in my experience if the patient is having symptoms they should be treated. It is known that cholesterol, low-density lipoprotein (LDL) and triglycerides are elevated in overt hypothyroidism. I have also treated many cases of subclinical hypothyroidism in which these levels have also been elevated. Also, cardiac function can improve significantly when subclinical hypothyroidism is treated. We are also finding some association with fibromyositis and sub-clinical hypothyroidism.

I find many patients have a family history of low thyroid. I believe that chlorine in our drinking and bathing water may be a major cause of low thyroid. Chlorine can actually replace the iodine in the thyroid molecule. Drugs such as Lithium and Cordarone can also cause low thyroid.

Estrogen use and pregnancy are associated with false elevations of total T4, whereas the use of salsalate, phenytoin sodium or high doses of aspirin or Phenobarbital may falsely lower total T4. Because drugs and hormones can affect the levels of T3 and T4, interpreting their results can be difficult at times. A formula has been developed to evaluate the levels of both, and the result is a T7 level that supposedly takes into consideration the different factors that influence T3 and T4 levels. Now the highly sensitive TSH (Thyroid Stimulating Hormone) level is being used. In most labs a TSH value over 5 means that you have low thyroid. The normal range is 0.4 to 5. If the TSH is below 2.8, it is probably sub-clinical low thyroid secondary to a *low functioning pituitary*. Recently some endocrinologists have recognized that a TSH between 3 and 5 should be suspect.

The pituitary gland, which is located beneath the brain in a pocket in the midline of the skull, secretes a hormone (TSH) that stimulates the thyroid to produce T4. The stimulated thyroid secretes the thyroid hormone T4 that circulates through the body and transforms into T3. T3 is four times more active on our metabolism than T4. Oftentimes I find patients who have a hard time converting T4 to T3. In these cases we have to treat them with T3 in addition to T4 or give them nutritional supplements to stimulate the body to convert the T4 to T3, especially if there is a vitamin, mineral or amino acid deficiency.

Many physicians use only synthetic T4 as a treatment (Synthroid being the most well known) because it can be produced in very exact doses and because they don't believe in natural supplements such as (Armour-Westhroid), which are not produced in such accurate doses. Armour and Westhroid contain both T3 and T4. So more hypothyroid cases can be benefited especially if the patient is T3-deficient and, in which case, they usually have more symptoms. I personally prefer Westhroid. However, I do use all supplements depending on the individual patient's needs. In addition to the history, examination and basal body temperature, I also use kinesiology to determine if and what thyroid or pituitary supplement a patient needs. I have treated hundreds of patients who were told by other physicians that their thyroid/pituitary function was normal and yet were markedly improved with treatment of their symptoms.

I have a list of thyroid symptoms that I have the patient review on every visit to determine if they have a problem and how it is progressing with treatment. Most doctors are overly afraid of treating a patient with thyroid disease because of possible side effects. They are primarily concerned about heart rhythm disorders and osteoporosis. Other than several cases of tachycardia (rapid heart rate) due to improper doses, I have not seen major side effects such as atrial fibrillation or heart attack.

I have not observed more osteoporosis compared to patients not on thyroid supplements. Of course I advise all my patients to take the proper supplements to prevent osteoporosis in addition to diet and increased exercise. The main supplements for preventing and treating osteoporosis are vitamin D3 or sunshine, boron, manganese, calcium, magnesium, zinc, copper, vitamin C, B vitamins and vitamin K, all of which are found in Osteo-B Plus. We used to think a high-protein diet accelerated osteoporosis, but this is now being questioned.

Symptoms possibly associated with thyroid disease are decreased immunity, increased infections, dry skin and hair, headache, poor memory, difficulty with concentration, mood swings, weight loss and weight gain, nervousness, depression, paranoid feelings, abdominal pain, constipation, irregular, heavy or painful menses, miscarriages, infertility, over-sensitivity to heat or cold, ringing of the ears and trouble with hearing, nightmares, sleep disturbances, loss of appetite, fatigue, low sexual desire, joint and/or muscle pain, increased blood pressure, heart palpitations, chest pain, and difficulty breathing, swelling in face or feet, brittle nails, hair loss, muscle weakness, dizziness, poor coordination, speech disturbances, dermatitis, tingling, burning or prickling of the skin, anemia, urinary frequency and decreased tendon reflexes.

Now I know the list is long, but since I have been semi-specializing in sub-clinical thyroid disease, I have found all of the above symptoms. Obviously, most patients present only a few symptoms; however, some patients present almost a majority of the possible symptoms. Since other conditions can present the same symptoms, the patient must be thoroughly evaluated. Don't allow yourself to be treated on the basis of laboratory work alone.

I believe I have greatly helped the majority of my patients by correctly diagnosing hypothyroidism and food allergies. Most physicians most frequently overlook these two conditions. The results are impressive and the patients are very grateful.

Other Medical Problems

There are other medical problems I frequently see and treat that many other physicians either ignore, fail to diagnose or don't believe exist. A list of short explanations should suffice, as there is considerable literature available on each of these subjects.

Chronic Fatigue Syndrome
It is unusual when I don't find an underlying problem to explain most of the symptoms such as systemic yeast infection, parasites, hypoglycemia, hypothyroidism, chronic virus infection, depression, heavy metal toxicity and hypoadrenalism, to name a few. Usually the patient has a low immune system as well.

Environmental Illness,
Multiple Food and Chemical Sensitivities
This is very often due to excessive pollution and is difficult to treat. Many physicians still do not accept this as a diagnosis; however, there is so much literature and confirming evidence that anyone who takes the time to investigate has to admit that it exists. I never heard of this before coming to Prescott, except for the food allergies.

Many people come here to live from all parts of the country because we have a relatively pollution-free environment. All of them have poorly functioning immune systems. Again, many have yeast, parasite, thyroid and hypoadrenal problems. They all must be detoxified and their underlying health problems corrected. Supplements that I have found very useful for these individuals are MSM, microhydrin and Transfer Factor to boost their immune system. Because of the resistance of many doctors to treating this condition, I have many patients who truly suffer from environment-related illnesses. Most have to live in specially designed living quarters. Various odors to which they are sensitive can cause them to be very ill. One patient of mine tapes around her doors at night to keep out odors of diesel and gasoline. Many doctors think these patients are "crazy" and indeed, many of them have anxiety, depression and other emotional problems. I believe that these emotional problems are secondary to the condition itself, rather than the emotional problems causing the patient to "think" they are sensitive to various odors such as chemicals or foods. This group of patients is usually the sickest (along with fibromyalgia) of any group.

Fibromyositis (Fibromyalgia)

Unfortunately, we are seeing more and more of this. This is a syndrome with many possible symptoms, the most prominent of which is muscular aches and pains with multiple tender localized and specific sites. Associated symptoms can be extreme fatigue, stiffness, depression and low sex drive. The cause of fibromyositis is unknown, but I suspect a viral or toxic chemical etiology and am currently investigating these possibilities. We are now using darkfield (live blood cell) analysis and are finding a "grub-like" parasite in the red blood cells of all fibromyalgic patients we have studied. There are many books on fibromyalgia, but to my knowledge none have identified a definite cause of the painful crippling condition. Another cause may be parasitic and/or mycoplasma infection. We are seeing much more of this in recent years, suggesting that it could also be related to environmental "poisons." Cervical spine dislocations could also be an important factor to be considered.

Fibromyalgia is very difficult to treat. Some patients respond to magnesium, malic acid, MSM, aromatherapy and gluconutrients. Others respond only to antidepressants and anti-inflammatories. I am currently experimenting with colostrum, fibrolytic pancreatic enzymes, Beta Glucans, and energy medicine in some of my patients to improve their immune system. The newest method I am trying is a microcurrent machine that was just approved for use by the FDA in November 1999. I also believe that eliminating allergy with NAET technique may be very beneficial. It appears that persons with fibromyalgia have a frequency consistent with multiple sclerosis made worse with sugar and artificial sweeteners. Recently here in Arizona, homeopathic physicians have been given a grant to study the effects of homeopathic remedies on fibromyalgia.

Hypoglycemia

Glucose tolerance tests will usually substantiate the diagnosis. Frequent feedings of protein and complex carbohydrates and avoidance of simple carbohydrates is necessary. Often, supplemental minerals such as chromium and/or vanadium are very helpful. It can be very simple to diagnose with kinesiology and history.

Systemic Candida (systemic fungal mycelial rhizoid)

This condition is due to common yeast turning into a different form: fungi (like a caterpillar turning into a moth), which invades the gut wall and then travels to all parts of the body, with resultant multiple symptoms. Often it does not respond well to prescription medication and in most cases will respond well to alternative medications. I have found that an oregano extract is very efficient in clearing the fungus in most cases. All of us have benign candida in our body. It has to turn into the fungal mycelial form before it becomes disease-producing. It can cause many symptoms. A number of books are available on this subject. Antibiotics, a poor diet and pH changes in your body can trigger the change from yeast to fungus.

Parasites

We all have them but not all of them cause us problems. They can also produce many symptoms: weight gain, weight loss, diarrhea, constipation, abdominal pain, skin rashes, cough, itching, arthritis, hypoglycemia, lowered immune system, fatigue, memory loss, blurred vision, and so on and so forth.
Unfortunately, unless a laboratory does testing that specializes in parasites, most of the time the diagnosis will be missed. Current laboratory testing finds only a small percent of the more than 1000 parasites that can live in your body. We have both prescription and alternative therapies. Parasites can inhabit muscle tissue, the digestive tract, the blood stream, the brain, and all other vital organs. We have found that the best method to diagnose parasite infestation is kinesiology and dark-field live-blood analysis. The usual method of diagnosing parasites is by stool exam, but even the most expert will miss many cases. I find that kinesiology is a very accurate method for diagnosing parasites. The tip of the finger (neutral) placed at a point midway between the umbilicus (belly button) and the iliac crest (left hip) will cause the arm to weaken if parasites are present. I recently found that drinking 8-15 drops of Miracle II Soap on an empty stomach will eliminate parasites if taken for a sufficient period of time (Miracle II, created by Clayton Tedeton, may be found at www.miracleii.net)

Dr. Frank Nova, Chief of the Laboratory for Parasitic Diseases at the National Institutes of Health, claims, "In terms of number, there are more parasitic infections acquired in this country than in Africa." Parasites can be contracted by eating unclean raw vegetables, drinking infected water, and by eating uncooked meat, especially pork and fish. They can also be acquired from animals. I see more parasite infections in the winter months. This may be due to eating vegetables that are shipped here from Mexico where parasites seem to be more prevalent.

Of interest to me is the fact that in all cases of cancer and fibromyalgia, I find that the patient also has a parasitic infestation. Only one time did I find a cancer patient who didn't have a parasite and when I told her that, she laughed and said she had just been treated and cleared of her parasites. I believe the parasitic infection lowers the patient's immune system and makes a person more likely to develop cancer. I believe that to improve a patient's likelihood of clearing cancer, the first thing that has to be considered is improving their immune system. This means to me that the parasites have to be eliminated first and foremost along with surgery, if that is indicated. I do not usually like chemotherapy, as I feel it tends to suppress the immune system, although I have used it in the past with good success in very selected cases. I feel that radiation when carefully given has less of an effect on the immune system than chemotherapy.

Hormone Replacement Therapy (HRT)

Much has been written on the benefits of HRT for improvement of menopause symptoms, heart disease, osteoporosis and stroke prevention. There is no question in my mind that HRT has merit in these conditions; however, I believe that natural hormones are much the better choice for most patients. Using kinesiology I determine what a patient best tests for—Premarin (from a pregnant horse's urine) or a more natural substance. There are three estrogens produced in a woman's body—estriol, estrone and estradiol.

Two of the hormones (estrone and estradiol) have been linked to increased risk of cancer, while estriol has been shown to be somewhat of a factor in preventing cancer. I prefer the use of Triestrogen, which contains eighty percent estriol, ten percent estrone and ten percent estradiol. Dr. Wright formulated it. It is a natural estrogen that has to be "compounded" by a compounding pharmacist and requires a prescription. It comes in varying strengths, and usually a 2.5 milligram dose is equivalent to 1.25 milligrams of Premarin.

I also prefer natural progesterone. Dr. John Lee has written extensively regarding this product. The brand that I find tests best (with kinesiology) is Progest. The dosage is determined by how fast it is absorbed. If it is absorbed rapidly after rubbing it on the skin (less than three minutes), I recommend that the cream be applied twice a day, usually to the abdominal wall. The commonly prescribed synthetic product "Provera" has many side effects of which the following are examples: Menstrual irregularities, dermatitis, depression, insomnia, nausea, jaundice, weight change, headache, dizziness, anxiety (to name a few!).

Natural Testosterone, DHEA and L-arginine all naturally improve a man's ability to have an erection, improve wound healing and help maintain strong heart muscles. Some women also need testosterone therapy.

Recently, some of the "good" effects of HRT have been questioned by some medical researchers. So time will tell. Maybe HRT needs to be reevaluated.

Chapter 4

The Mind

We are on the threshold of a new paradigm—one in which energy and frequencies are both understood to play a role in consciousness and health. The subtle, invisible forces that make up our world have been there all along, but they're just beginning to be recognized.

Law of the Harvest

It is plainly explained in the Bible but most people do not realize the implications of the "Law of The Harvest." Consider your mind, that in all of its ramifications is your garden, and your thoughts are the seeds. What you plant you shall reap. When you plant a kernel of corn you expect to raise corn. You don't expect to grow potatoes or cherries. You also expect this kernel of corn to grow into a plant that will produce several ears of corn with many kernels. The seed has to be planted in the proper type of soil. You cannot plant on barren ground and expect to harvest a bountiful crop. You know that if you carefully tend to this corn plant, weed, nurture and water it, the crop provides a better yield.

Now, look at the effects of our thoughts. Remember that our thoughts are as seeds and our mind is the garden. If you plant positive seeds in your garden and nurture them, they will yield positive results. If you plant negative thoughts, you will grow negative results. We can determine our future by what we think of today. Thinking positive thoughts will result in the development of positive actions and deeds.

I've been told, "Well, I've been thinking positively for several months now and I haven't noticed any positive results." This may be true. One important aspect of the Law of the Harvest has been forgotten. Different seeds grow to fruition at different times. In general, weeds mature much quicker than many of the plants we like to grow. Thinking positively results in some thoughts maturing more rapidly than others. For example, in my garden I plant radishes and corn at the same time. The radishes are ready to eat long before the corn. Some thoughts are like oak trees. If you plant an acorn, it takes a very long time for an oak tree to grow and produce acorns. So then our thoughts, even though they're positive, may take a long time to mature. We must not lose sight of the individuality of our thoughts.

I often tell my patients, "Your symptoms are due to anxiety and stress." "But I'm not anxious and I'm not stressed," is often the response. "Well, when were you anxious and stressed? Was it a week, a month, or a year ago?" It sometimes takes that long for stress to develop into a symptom. We must be aware of the time relationship between the planting of the seed and the moment it bears fruit.

You can change your future by the way you think today. Don't delay, take the necessary steps to have a better, brighter, healthier, wealthier future by putting the proper seeds into your mental garden now. Phrase the mental suggestions very carefully. Nurture them by thinking of them repeatedly. Faith is an important element of positive thinking. Faith can be thought of as planting the seed in the right soil; if you don't have faith it's like throwing the seed on barren ground. Desire is the energy that helps positive thoughts grow. Desire is like sunlight. The stronger the desire and the more sustained it is, the more certain that the result will be realized. Act as though your positive thoughts have already been granted. Everything in the world originated with a thought. Every wish begins with a thought, and if your thoughts flow in the same direction as your faith and desire, these wishes will be realized.

Discipline will also help your garden grow. Discipline is necessary to plant the garden properly, to nourish it, to water and weed it, and to harvest the crop. Without discipline you will not have success in thinking positive thoughts. You have to plant the ideas properly and persevere in your thoughts and actions. If you do not actively tend to your garden, it will not grow well and you will not reap a harvest. Unfortunately, the negative things we plant require very little nurturing and seem to grow without much effort.

Negative thoughts are nourished by what we observe in everyday life: what we hear on the news; what we see on television and in the movies; what others tell us. Negativity is abundant, and we tend to absorb it without realizing it. Weed out the negative thoughts. Every night before you go to sleep, review your day's activities and thoughts. Mentally weed out any negative thoughts and replace them with positive ones for tomorrow. Develop a positive plan of action. With this accomplished, your subconscious mind can act on your positive thoughts, thus helping guarantee a bountiful harvest.

There are several things that will diminish your garden's productivity. Doubt diminishes your abilities. Think positive and look at the good side of things. There is a good side to everything; the trick is finding it. One of my mothers favorite sayings was, "It's an ill wind that doesn't blow some good." Always look for the good in things and avoid focusing on the possible bad effects.

Fear is like a fence, it doesn't let you go where you would like. "The greater the fear, the higher the fence." Fear is a negative emotion and must not be allowed into your mental garden. It is a deterrent to what you need to accomplish. When you become fearful, relax, breathe deeply, think positively and try to transplant the fear in your mind with confidence and faith. Winston Churchill once said, "The only thing we have to fear is fear itself." I've always felt close to Winston inasmuch as our birthdays were the same, except for the year!

Psychic Abilities (Intuition)

Alan Sandage, seventy-five, a noted scientist and astronomer, had been an atheist most of his life. He finally accepted God at the age of fifty. His statement expresses my views as well: "It was my science that drove me to the conclusion the world is much more complicated than can be explained by science. It is only through the supernatural I can understand the mystery of existence."

In the last forty to fifty years, many people have been greatly interested in exploring the wonders of outer space. While, on the other hand, I have been more curious about "inner space," the ability of the mind to control the body. The subconscious mind controls all body functions without verbal directions. You do not have to think to breathe or make your heart beat. The power of the subconscious mind makes hypnosis a valuable therapeutic tool.

It has been my experience that science and religion are often very much opposed to each other. However, with more understanding of the universe, the cosmos, outer space and our subconscious mind's abilities, it appears to me that the two are coming closer together. The more we learn about these entities, the closer science and spirituality will become.

A few anecdotes will illustrate my point. While I was in the Air Force I learned to use the "pendulum technique" to test and question the subconscious. The technique consists of holding a string with a weighted object at the far end. The movement of the weight provides a yes or no answer to the question. You will receive an answer to whatever you properly ask of your subconscious.

Numerous military personnel asked me when and where they might be transferred. I was remarkably accurate. In the late summer, I began to think about baseball and the World Series. I used the "pendulum" to determine which team was going to win, hoping it would be my favorite team—the Detroit Tigers. Unfortunately, the pendulum indicated that it would be the Boston Red Sox. When I checked the standings I saw the Red Sox were in sixth place. I figured the pendulum was wrong; however, I recorded the observation as I did on most of my readings. Several months later I observed that the Red Sox had surged from sixth place to first place.

Over several years, my overall prediction rate using the pendulum was approximately eighty-two percent. This impressed me tremendously, since these predictions were not responses to simple yes and no questions. These predictions and questions had many possible answers. They were not constructed for simple yes and no responses. They could not be explained on the basis of chance. During this time, I would mentally ask people to call me in five minutes or to write me a letter within a week. The vast majority of the time, these requests were fulfilled. I no longer use the pendulum method. I do comparable testing on my patients utilizing kinesiology.

During the Christmas season a lovely Scottish lady worked as a Red Cross volunteer. We spoke briefly about the Officer's Christmas party. The following day she planned to shop for a party dress. I closed my eyes and saw what I thought was a beautiful dress. I described it to her. She doubted if there was anything like I had described in the town of Grand Forks. So I closed my eyes again and visualized the letters S E A R. I asked her to looked for a store with the letters S E A R but not Sears. Not being familiar with the stores in Grand forks, I had no idea what the search would entail. Two days later she told me the following story. She went to Grand Forks as I had suggested. She found a store by the name of SEARBYS and went in and asked for the dress I'd described. Much to her amazement, they brought it out. She spent the rest of the day looking through other stores in Grand Forks for a similar dress but could not find one. She returned to the first store, bought the dress and wore it to the Christmas dance.

A different type of psychic ability manifested itself during my last six months at Grand Forks Air Force Base. I found that while I was talking to someone on the telephone, I could close my eyes and visualize the person, their surroundings, how they were dressed and the contents of the entire room. This ability lasted for only six months. I do not know how I acquired or lost this ability, but it would be nice if it returned.

Many cells in our body are able to produce chemicals and enzymes that mimic other organs. When we say we have a "gut feeling," we are in essence saying that our stomach is thinking for us. When we say we "have a heartache," we are likely describing an emotional condition.

A book was recently written about the post-operative experiences of heart-transplant patients. It appears that people receiving organ transplants often assume personality traits of the donor. One story in the book described a girl who received a heart from another young girl who had been murdered. After a time, the girl began having specific feelings and dreams and was evaluated by a psychologist. She was able to give details of the murder that was not previously known. Most importantly, she was able to provide information that led to the identification and conviction of the killer.

We are just beginning to understand that our body is a complex mixture of chemical molecules. Each time we learn something new about the body it's like reading a new chapter in a book. Edgar Cayce would go into a trance and determine the diagnosis and proper treatment for people who were many miles away. There are numerous books written about Edgar Cayce the prophet. If you have not read any of them, I recommend that you do so. I always thought how wonderful it would be if I could diagnose people miles away.

While interning at Borgess's Hospital in Kalamazoo, I was called to Detroit for an Army induction physical. I thought the request was unusual because I'd been classified 4-Fdue to two serious bouts of hepatitis while in college. The Army, however, wanted to re-examine me. On the way, I determined to prove to myself if mental telepathy could work. I started sending mental messages to a friend in Detroit whom I hadn't talked to in six months. I suggested that she meet me at the Greyhound Bus Station. I knew if she got the message it would be due to mental telepathy, as she had no other way of knowing I was coming to Detroit.

When I got to the station, I looked for her; however, she did not show up. I waited for about half an hour. When she didn't appear, I assumed that my mental telepathy experiment had failed. I walked two blocks to the hotel, and much to my amazement my friend was waiting for me in the lobby. Over a cup of coffee I told her what I had been attempting to do and asked her how she knew I would be in Detroit. She related that she had a strong feeling about me earlier in the morning that quickly became an obsession. Not understanding the situation, she called my wife and asked about my whereabouts. She was told I was on my way to Detroit for the examination as well as the name of my hotel.

She came to the hotel to ascertain what had prompted her sudden impulse to contact me. I have never seen her since.

My wife had the misfortune of losing her diamond wedding ring set while peeling potatoes. She had placed them on some paper with the peels, and unknowingly a houseguest threw them in the garbage. Priceless trash indeed! That afternoon we took a drive to look at antelope roaming around the Prescott countryside. My wife noticed she did not have her rings. We realized what had happened and hurried back to town. The garbage man came on Thursdays and we had to get back before he picked up the trash. Unfortunately, we were too late and my wife was devastated. For three years she searched the house, inside and out, hoping we had been wrong about the rings being thrown out with the potato peelings. She was so distraught that she couldn't watch a diamond advertisement on the T.V. without crying.

One day while talking to a patient about mental powers, she mentioned that she was a spiritualist. I told her my aunt also practiced spiritualism. She gave me a small book to read on the subject. Included was a description of the materialization of lost objects. After reading this I remembered that I had lost a ring playing softball many years earlier. The game was stopped and both teams looked in vain for the ring. I then tried to materialize the ring. Two weeks later, I opened my son's closet door and the lost ring was sitting on the sill.

Recalling this event, I thought materialization might help me again. I concentrated on having her rings come back for her birthday, May 13th. I told no one of my efforts. Two days before her birthday she called, crying for joy, because her rings had returned! After I told her they were not to come back until her birthday she got very upset thinking that maybe I had been hiding the rings for three years. I told her that I was very busy and I'd give her a complete explanation when I got home.

When I arrived home that evening, she joyfully described the events surrounding the discovery of her rings. She was in the upstairs bathroom washing her hands when she heard something fall to the floor in the adjoining walk-in closet. To her amazement she found the diamond ring on the floor, as if it had dropped from the sky. She started crying and thanking God. Her mother and friends rejoiced at her good fortune.

Later, before I returned home, she was washing the ring, which was very dirty, and reflecting wistfully on the still missing part of the wedding ring set. Returning to the walk-in closet, she found the wedding ring in the same place her diamond ring had been earlier. I explained to her what I had done in an attempt to retrieve her rings. To this day, we both are very thankful for their return.

Soon after this episode I increased my efforts in kinesiology. In so doing, my intuitive ability seemed to re-grow. I aggressively tested my patients for various allergic reactions. The substances I used came in vials. I would have the patient hold them in their outstretched arm. If the arm went weak, I knew they were sensitive and must avoid the food product, chemical, vitamin supplement, and so on. After several years of such testing I could tell the results beforehand. I found that by reading a list of ingredients and focusing on my patients, I could determine their sensitivities. To test myself I would use kinesiology for each substance. Proudly, I was correct each time.

My intuitive abilities have been refined to the point at which I use only a list of ingredients to review for allergic sensitivity. This saves time and money. With patient compliance and appropriate testing, my findings lead to successful treatment regimens. I use this approach for compatibility with medications and supplements.

I've also found that I can mentally question a person about their health and receive a correct answer whether I am sitting next to them, across the room, talking to them on the telephone or whether I just know their name and address. I practiced this telepathic method of diagnosis by asking friends or patients if they knew someone who had major illnesses. They would then give me their names and addresses, very much like Edgar Cayce, and I would be able to consistently (but not one-hundred percent of the time) determine the proper diagnosis.

I get many calls from all over the United States and Canada from people who ask me to diagnose their illness and recommend treatment options. I've been very successful; however, I cannot make a diagnosis without first mentally focusing on the person. I evaluate the body and concentrate on different illnesses as I go through each organ system. I cannot simply obtain a person's name and address and instantaneously provide a diagnosis. I must mentally examine each body system and ask specific mental questions of the individual to get a valid diagnosis.

A friend's mother had been sick for several years. She'd been treated by numerous physicians with little relief of her many symptoms. I asked my friend to have his mother call me. While talking with her, I went through the process I just described and determined that her primary problem was food allergy. I told her which foods to avoid and within a month her symptoms had totally cleared. She was so impressed that her husband called me about several of his conditions. After arriving at a diagnosis, the treatment plan provided excellent results. This couple subsequently traveled from Florida to my office in Prescott for a hands-on examination.

While on vacation another friend called about his daughter, who was having jaw pain when she chewed. This was the only time it seemed to bother her. My first clinical impression was that she had a temporal mandibular joint (TMJ) syndrome. To be certain, I suggested trying the absentee (intuitive) kinesiology method. Afterwards, I told him it was not TMJ but rather an abscessed tooth. My friend didn't agree because his daughter didn't have a toothache. I suggested they go to the dentist anyway. The next day he called to tell me that the dentist did indeed remove an abscessed tooth and her symptoms had cleared.

Several years ago I had my oldest daughter give me the names of people she knew with illnesses. I would then give her my intuitive diagnoses. In one case, I told her the person had advanced arthritis, which was true, but I also told her that he had heart disease. She said, "Well, dad, you're wrong on that one. His heart is fine as far as I know. He doesn't have any heart problems." I said, "Oh, well, I can make mistakes as well as anyone else—that's why they put erasers on pencils." A few months ago she reminded me about the patient who had arthritis and whom I claimed had heart disease. She said I was right all along. He recently underwent quadruple bypass heart surgery.

I tell you these stories to demonstrate the power of the mind over physical matters. I want you to realize that these abilities exist, not just for me but also to some degree for anyone with the right amount of mental conditioning, belief and effort. I firmly believe that intuition is everyone's sixth sense, along with hearing, seeing, feeling, tasting and smelling. With future generations the mind's abilities will become widely accepted and used on a daily basis.

There are an increasing number of alternative practitioners in the United States. The theories of alternative medicine are being widely discussed and even studied at the National Institutes of Health. It is my fervent desire to further the development and application of techniques not currently in vogue with the allopathic establishment.

My intuitive or psychic abilities are presently limited to medical diagnoses and treatment. Regrettably, I do not seem to have any psychic abilities in any other area. I am very poor at making investment decisions and could surely use some intuition in these matters! Perhaps I should have listened to my son, Stephen, some twenty years ago when he was seven and he said, "Dad, why don't you just decide what to do with your investments and then do the opposite?" Had I followed his advice I would be in much better financial condition. However, I'm happy, we eat regular meals and I thank God every day to be alive and see the sun come up and be able to give service to my patients.

I've been told that intuitive evaluation and kinesiology are the devil's work. I do not believe this for a moment. Anything that helps people and is done with good intentions is a gift from the Lord. In fact, I have become much more spiritual in my Christian beliefs because of the gifts I've been given. There is no question in my mind that the Lord God allows us free choice. I choose to live by three rules I share with my patients, regardless of their illness. *Love everyone, forgive everyone*, and *don't judge*. I'll continue to repeat this credo until it sinks into everyone's head. These are the basics for good health and enjoyable living.

We have been told, "Ask and it shall be given unto you." This I have done. Regarding my intuitive abilities, I have sought them, asked to have them given to me and it appears that I have been blessed with this ability. I try to get my patients to understand that their bodies are literally temples of God. As such, we should take care of them in the best way possible.

At the present time I am accepting phone calls from people in the United States, Canada and Europe who ask that I diagnose and suggest treatment programs for them. I am more than happy to do this, as I have been able to help many who have not been able to get medical help from others. I do not charge for this service; however, I do accept donations from those who feel I have provided them with an accurate diagnosis and treatment program that has given them relief of their symptoms. Information regarding times I am available for consultations can be obtained by calling my office at (928) 717-0678. All donations will be used to help establish my thirty-year dream of a holistic medical clinic, that is, the "Rainbow Medicine Lodge."

Hypnotherapy

There are many theories regarding hypnosis. In truth, no one completely understands why or how it works. Experts often describe hypnosis as an altered state of consciousness. It is a natural state, every bit as natural as being asleep or being awake. We all experience spontaneous hypnotic states every day of our lives, such as arriving at your destination without any recollection of the details of the trip or fantasizing while watching flames flicker in the fireplace. Oftentimes an individual must be called several times before letting go of the subject of their hypnosis, such as a movie, a book, and so forth. All are hypnotic events occurring spontaneously in your day.

Another way to look at hypnosis is to see it as a procedure with which the hypnotist communicates with your subconscious. Habits, both good and bad, reside in the subconscious mind. In order to establish new constructive habits such as developing a positive outlook on events in our lives or to eliminate old destructive ones such as smoking or overeating, it is necessary to communicate with the subconscious mind. Our subconscious mind doesn't know the difference between good and bad, or truth and fiction. The subconscious accepts everything it receives. It's extremely important that we store positive thoughts in the subconscious, even if we have to lie about it! Positive thoughts will become reality with emphasis. Conversely, if you allow your subconscious to entertain fearful thoughts, hatred or lack of self-confidence, your personality will reflect these attitudes.

With hypnosis, the individual follows the suggestion of the hypnotist or acts on autosuggestion. By repeating these thoughts long enough, they will turn into acts and concrete tangible realities will evidence themselves. To get the best results with hypnosis, the idea to be communicated must be clear, repeated, and prolonged to achieve the best effect. I have found that some people are better transmitters than receivers and vice versa. Remember, everyone is unique. Everyone has special talents that they have developed or can develop. We also have numerous abilities we've failed to recognize and improve upon.

People are often afraid that a person will make them quack like a duck or reveal some personal secret while under hypnosis. This is only done in sideshows, fairs, and so forth, and has no place in medical treatment. Remember, you cannot be compelled to do something under hypnosis that you would not do in a normal state of mind.

Early in this century there was heated debate on this subject. One night at a well-known convention hall, two competing hypnotists decided to settle the question once and for all. The first hypnotist strongly felt he could not get a person to do anything he did not want to do. Under hypnosis, the volunteer from the audience was told to go and steal from someone in the crowd. The person refused. The hypnotist was elated and claimed that he had proved his point. The second hypnotist told the same volunteer to take money from the rich people in the audience and give it to the poor. With this suggestion, the subject left the stage and promptly took money from numerous individuals in the gathering. The second hypnotist felt vindicated.

Both claimed victory because of the structure of their hypnotic suggestions. If a hypnotist told a subject to take off their clothes, they probably would not comply. However, if the same person were told he was tired, he probably would undress for bed. Make sure you have a very reliable hypnotist if you decide to use hypnosis as a therapy. It can be very rewarding for those who use it wisely.

We are constantly influenced by people we meet; friends, relatives, and so on, just as our environment influences us. You may have noticed, for example, that when you are around nervous people you become nervous. You are unknowingly receiving the other person's vibrations and it has an effect on you. The mind has an all-powerful control over matter. This control can extend to the bodies and minds of *other* people. You are a product of what you think and also of what you eat, how you exercise, and so forth. There are many diseases that doctors presently believe are psychosomatic. The diseases are initiated by the patient's own thought processes.

I first observed the power of hypnosis when a young girl with a severely lacerated tongue was sutured under hypnosis without the slightest discomfort or anxiety. I became fascinated with the ability to direct the subconscious mind to control and aid our bodies. It was not until eight years later, while serving in the Air Force at Grand Forks, North Dakota, that I began employing hypnotic techniques to reduce the suffering of my patients. Hypnosis is a very effective and powerful modality. The following are a few of the many experiences I have had with the hypnotic technique.

An airman came to the office one morning wanting narcotics for headaches. After a thorough examination, I refused to write a prescription. He became quite upset, claiming he'd been on narcotics for several years. I asked him if I could use hypnosis to wean him off the narcotics. He stated that several people had tried unsuccessfully to hypnotize him. I implored him to give it another try. Over the next three weeks with approximately two hypnosis sessions a week, I was able to resolve his headaches and get him off the narcotics. I followed him closely. He had no further headaches or need for narcotics.

I regressed this airman to a previous lifetime in approximately 1861, in the Black Hills of South Dakota. Since I have been there myself, I quizzed him while he was in the regressed state on many points about the geography of the area. I asked him about the trees, terrain, gold prospecting, how to handle a muzzle-loader, and so forth. He was able to answer all these questions correctly. Without changing his hypnotic depth, I brought him back to the present. He was totally unable to answer the same questions. Since I was not a believer in reincarnation, this episode made me think more of the possibilities.

An Air Force wife had many phobias, and we cleared all of them with hypnosis except for the fear of water. Her husband attended most of the hypnotic sessions. After discussing the possibilities I regressed her back to the age of eighteen, when her phobia started. I methodically took her back to ages nineteen, eighteen, seventeen, sixteen, and fifteen. I could not find any reason for her fear. One day I regressed her to a previous lifetime and found that at the age of eighteen, she'd fallen from a boat in the ocean off the Florida coast. She became very hysterical. With hypnotic suggestion, she was able to calm down and regain her composure. Afterwards, she knew she had been very upset but was unaware of what she had experienced.

Several months passed, and I was still unable to get rid of her water phobia. I asked her if we could repeat her hypnotic session with some minor changes. She agreed, much to the delight of her husband and myself. On this occasion, I took her back to a lifetime in approximately 1628. I found that she had been born in Sweden. She had come to the "New World" with her parents. Both her parents had died enroute, leaving her alone. She was cared for by a lady she called the "Lady in Black." This person used her as somewhat of a slave. Subsequently, they traveled down the east coast of the United States and ended up on a boat off the coast of Florida, where she fell overboard and was drowned. Interestingly, she was not really upset by her drowning. What bothered her most was that no one on board had tried to save her. After obtaining all the information we needed, I gave her the proper post-hypnotic suggestions. Since discussing the facts of her past life, she has been symptom-free of her water phobia.

With more and more experience, hypnosis became much easier to perform. I successfully treated many different cases of depression, phobias, fears, cravings and addictions. I was also able to help patients with back pains, bursitis, headache and allergies.

I treated a young mother for a very severe case of pharyngitis. She was unable to swallow any fluids. She was dehydrated and very ill. I told her that she would need to be admitted to the hospital for intravenous fluids and medication. She had no one to take care of her children if she were hospitalized; therefore, I resorted to hypnosis. I told her that when she awoke from hypnosis, her throat would not be as sore and she would be able to swallow fluids. The soreness would persist on a lower scale until her throat infection healed. With these suggestions, she was immediately able to drink fluids and to take oral antibiotics and continued to do so until her throat was clear.

When I worked in the emergency room, an airman came in with an acute torticollis of the neck. This condition produces extremely painful spasms of the neck muscles. Normally, muscle relaxants and pain medications are used but with poor immediate results. Therefore, I elected to use hypnosis. Instead of using a relaxing, maternal type of induction, I decided on the command, autocratic type of induction. I thought it would be effective since I was a captain and he was a private. I commanded him to go under hypnosis. I further commanded that his neck spasms be resolved immediately. In less than five minutes his neck was supple and pain free.

A young, intelligent college girl had a history of epilepsy and marked depression. She had attempted suicide on many occasions and had been hospitalized in several mental institutions. She was on multiple anti-anxiety and antidepressant medicines in addition to antiseizure medication. Although she did not get along with her parents, they were very concerned about her. One day her mother, a practical nurse, asked me if I thought hypnosis might help her. I said there would be nothing lost in trying. The young girl was a good subject. Immediately after the first hypnosis session, she walked out to the waiting room, gave her mother a hug and told her she loved her. Mom was flabbergasted. In less than three months of treatment, the young woman no longer showed any signs of depression. She was off all medication, including her antiseizure medication.

In another case I was able to regress a female patient into three previous lifetimes. This girl was from the southeastern part of the United States and had a typical southern accent. When regressed to the lifetime spent in Ireland, she immediately spoke with an Irish brogue. During another hypnosis session, I theorized that if I could take a person back in time, why couldn't I take a person forward in time? I first took her a couple of years into the future, to about 1969, and asked her who the president was. She quickly answered that it was Richard Nixon. She was unhappy that he had been elected; she said he was elected by a small margin. I asked her the identity of the vice president. She took several moments before replying, "Spiro Agnew." I had never heard of him! A year and a half later, after the election, her visions were a reality.

In another session, I took her only a month into the future and asked her to read the Grand Forks newspaper. She told me that an attempted missile firing at the base had ended in failure. Later, the same afternoon, while sitting in the officer's lounge, a colonel sat down next to me who'd just arrived from Moffit Air

Force Base. He was attached to the missile squadron. I told him I heard there was going to be a test firing of a missile on a certain day. He became very agitated and jumped up from his chair. Since he was the only one on the base who knew about this missile firing, he thought there must be a security leak. He was further alarmed that such information was privy to a medical officer. He demanded to know how I got this information. After I told him how I knew, he calmed down but remained very skeptical. I couldn't help but add, "Don't worry, Jim, it's going to be a flop anyway."

We subsequently became very good friends. I would tell him ahead of time whether his missile firings would be good or bad. While in a progressive state, this patient was one-hundred percent accurate. These experiences further convinced me of the powers of the mind. In subsequent hypnosis sessions she saw a number of things, including people zooming around in air buggies in the year 2020. She described the air buggy as a small car that traveled on a cushion of air. These sessions were taped and are available to confirm these revelations.

While in the service, I did some moonlighting in a small Michigan town. With the permission of the Air Force, I worked there two nights a week and Saturdays. An elderly lady in her late seventies came to my office one day complaining of marked anxiety following an automobile accident. She was very much afraid to drive or ride in a car. The ability to drive was important because she had to go close to fifty miles in either direction to obtain medicine and other essential items. With only one hypnosis session, I was able to eliminate her fear of driving and riding in a car. Afterwards, she was able to use her car as she had before the accident.

I once treated an obstetrical nurse for weight loss. In one session she became "possessed." She started talking in the voice of an old British lady. This lady proceeded to tell me a number of things about myself. She chastised me for being too aggressive, and that before I went further with some of my alternative ideas, I should stop and heal myself. When she spoke, it literally shook me to the core. A friend of mine witnessed this session with guarded curiosity. When the entity left, we proceeded with the weight loss session. Every time I listen to the tape, I get the "heebie-jeebies." Perhaps because of the need to heal myself, I lost most of my psychic (intuitive) abilities for over ten years.

Hypnosis can be a very powerful alternative method of treatment for many conditions. It is paramount that you have someone hypnotize you whom you trust implicitly. If you're receiving any type of medical therapy, you must have a therapist who is knowledgeable both from a medicinal and psychological standpoint.

Self-Hypnosis

The subconscious mind is very selective in how it accepts suggestions. Take a person who tends to be excessively hungry. You might be tempted to direct your subconscious with the thought, "I am not hungry, I am not hungry." Unfortunately, this type of suggestion to the subconscious will not work. The subconscious will not focus on the words "*I am not, I am not,*" but will instead be influenced by the word "*hungry.*" A person using this particular type of command to the subconscious will oftentimes only aggravate his hunger symptoms. A more proper way of presenting this suggestion would be to say: "I am easily satisfied with small amounts of food."

In the following autosuggestion, "I will not be angry any longer," the word angry will be picked up by the mind. This may aggravate your problem. It would be better to reword the suggestion to: "From now on I'm going to be happy, healthy and contented." Positive suggestions are essential.

Let me give you a simple outline for self-hypnosis. First, when practicing or studying self-hypnosis (autosuggestion), select a time of day when you are relaxed and don't have too much on your mind. It's important to have time to relax. Pick a place where it's quiet and the lighting is subdued. If you like, you may include background music. Try to avoid outside noises and other distractions. Make yourself comfortable; a loose-fitting robe is probably the best.

Now, sit in a chair. Don't lie down when you first begin doing self-hypnosis. If you get too relaxed, you could fall asleep and interfere with the hypnotic process. Place your hands in your lap, palms down, and take deep breaths. Make sure that you breathe in slowly and let it out slowly over and over again. Let yourself become limp and relaxed. Focus your eyes on a particular object. It doesn't matter what the object is. It can be a picture, a candle, or a light. An object above eye level is best.

After focusing on the object for some time, tell yourself that your eyes are becoming tired. Keep repeating the words, "rest and relax" to yourself, and your eyes will become more tired. The eyelids will become fatigued and eventually when they want to close, let them. After your eyes close, concentrate on something. The subject is not important. It could be the pendulum on an old clock swinging back and forth, a seascape or whatever is pleasant to you. It doesn't matter what you picture, although I find it more effective if I focus on something monotonous.

As you relax further, imagine yourself doing something you enjoy such as fishing, reading, walking along a path in a flower garden or lying on a sun-drenched beach. Visualize yourself in the activity. Hear the sounds. Take in the aromas. You must constantly remind yourself to rest and relax. You are in control. When you are sufficiently relaxed, give yourself the suggestions you prepared beforehand. Repeating the suggestions, like reminding yourself to rest and relax, is very important. Practice the same way each time. Changing methods will interfere with the process. When you want to terminate the session, tell yourself you will wake alert and refreshed, and then count to three and open your eyes.

After several practice sessions the hypnotic state will be easier to achieve. You will be able to hear things going on around you while performing self-hypnosis. You may hear the birds singing in the trees or waves lapping on the shore.

It is necessary to practice self-hypnosis ten to twenty minutes per day. The more you practice, the quicker and better will be the results. Initially, you may not experience deep hypnosis. Pretend you are under, and go through the entire procedure as if you actually were hypnotized. Practice giving yourself the post-hypnotic suggestions you want to achieve. You can give these during the course of hypnosis, and you can also be very specific in giving post-hypnotic suggestions just prior to awakening.

Certain basic post-hypnotic suggestions should be given in addition to your own specific suggestions. Tell yourself you will feel alert and refreshed when you wake. If you are practicing self-hypnosis before bedtime, tell yourself that you are ready to sleep and will awaken completely rested. Tell yourself that you will be healthy. Tell yourself that whenever you repeat the words "rest and relax," it will enable you to go under hypnosis very quickly and easily. Finally, give yourself the same specific suggestions as when you were relaxed.

Self-hypnosis can be a wonderful tool to maintain and improve your health. There is nothing to fear with this technique. There is no way that you can harm yourself with self-hypnosis as long as you think positively.

Rest and relax, focus, be positive.

Rest and relax, focus, be positive.

Rest and relax, focus, be positive.

Rest and relax, focus, be positive.

Rest and relax, focus, be positive.

Thought Field Therapy

Early in 1998 one of my closest friends, a healer in his own right, told me about a new technique he learned called *thought field therapy*. Dr. Roger Callahan, a graduate of my alma mater, the University of Michigan, originated this protocol. The treatment consists of sequential tapping of acupuncture meridians in a precise serial fashion. The sequence of the tapping is determined by the condition and kinesiology.

Dr. Callahan has treated thousands of cases with this worldwide technique. He specializes in addictions, phobias and depressions. He has achieved many actual cures and not just temporary alleviation of the symptoms. Due to his success, Dr. Callahan decided to devote his efforts to teaching his technique to others.

I sent for the original tapes and reviewed them thoroughly. Before I attended a course seminar in Indian Wells, California, a patient called me from Phoenix in the midst of a panic attack wanting some tranquilizers. Using my intuitive kinesiology, I told her where to tap and within minutes her anxiety was alleviated without any medication.

During the course, Dr. Callahan discussed a patient he had treated for years for hydrophobia with minimal success. He administered thought field therapy and after one treatment she lost her fear of water without any reoccurrence. After thousands of cases, Dr. Callahan developed algorithms that work on a majority of his patients for each specific problem. However, I have found that treating each person individually provides better results.

Dr. Callahan's students around the world can call him, or one of his students with advanced training, for help with difficult cases. By recording the patient's voice on a special machine, they can analyze the voice tracing and determine what meridian should be tapped and in what sequence. I was very impressed with Dr. Callahan and his gift of training people in the use of thought field therapy.

Returning to my office, I combined Dr. Callahan's principles with my intuitive ability to develop what I term intuitive thought field therapy. I have achieved excellent results with every patient treated with this approach, including those I see in the office and others that I administer to over the telephone.

As previously mentioned, the tapping sequence is of utmost importance. Each condition has its own serial sets of tapping. I like to call them recipes. Each recipe is different. You cannot usually use one person's recipe to treat another.

I give each patient a recipe they can follow at home to resolve their symptoms. One of the first cases of major depression I treated in this manner involved a woman who had been depressed for over forty years due to the loss of loved ones. Within eight minutes, her depression was gone, and to my knowledge it has not returned.

Several weeks ago, a lady called from Illinois threatening to commit suicide. I used intuitive thought field therapy over the phone and she immediately felt much better. She asked how much I charged. I told her that I didn't charge for phone consultations; however, she was so pleased with the results that she sent a check anyway.

Last week, a patient with severe depression desperately needed some antidepressants. After testing him with kinesiology for various anti-depressants, I wrote a prescription but asked him to try thought field therapy first. I described the technique. He agreed to participate even though he was certain it would not work. Upon completing the session, he experienced immediate relief of his depression. I don't mean after five or ten minutes but *immediately.* I could see that he was feeling much better, smiling and joking with me. He said he felt much better but still didn't believe thought field therapy had caused the results. I told him to go home and see how he felt for the next couple of days. If the symptoms returned, he was to call me and get the prescription filled. He subsequently stopped by the office. I said, "It appears you're still feeling better. He replied, "Yes, I certainly am, but I still don't believe in it." This is a good example of how this technique can work whether a person believes in it or not.

A daughter of a good friend came to my home crying so hard she couldn't stop. I spent most of the day talking with her and inquiring about her history. I found she had numerous problems. In the evening, I elected to do thought field therapy for depression and for self-hatred. Afterward, I told the young lady to get a good night's sleep and promised that she would feel better in the morning. She doubted she would get any sleep and was certain that she would not feel better in the morning. The next morning she was radiant and smiling, exclaiming that she'd had a wonderful night's sleep.

She spent the next few days with us, and at no time was she depressed. We worked on a number of her other problems with thought field therapy. When she left, she was a totally different person, and a better person. She was given "recipes" to use at home should the need arise.

I have closely followed most of my thought field therapy cases to determine whether or not the effects are long-lasting. Patients can experience a psychological reversal if they are exposed to something to which they are sensitive. This may be a specific food, drink or odor such as the outgassing of a detergent in their clothes. Patients must be instructed on keeping a diary to help determine what might be reversing them. Patients who have had psychological reversals can often reverse them by simple tapping of the outside of their hand. This is the small intestine meridian. There are also other areas that can be tapped in specialized cases.

Dr. Royal Fuller, of Las Vegas, has been using thought field therapy in conjunction with a pre- and post-treatment machine that records the status of the autonomic nervous system. He has found that after proper treatment with thought field therapy, the autonomic nervous system returns to normal very quickly. This is very impressive because he is able to graphically record the results. In addition to the patient's testimony regarding his progress, Dr. Fuller can actually compare before and after graphs demonstrating autonomic improvement.

I suspect there will be increased fear, anxiety, depression and even terror in the coming millennium, which will require physicians to utilize additional treatment modalities such as thought field therapy.

Chapter 5

Path to Better Health

There are many extraordinary therapies on the path to better health. They form a sound foundation in the field of holistic medicine and can help us reclaim basic health and healing that have been forgotten in our culture.

Kinesiology

George Goodhart, D.C., a pioneer in the field of muscle testing, described his technique as *applied kinesiology*. I was introduced to kinesiology in 1969 at a lecture given by Dr. Bruce West. The hall was packed. When I saw what he was doing, I stood up and called him a charlatan. I just couldn't believe that it was possible. He invited me to the stage and proceeded to demonstrate responses nothing short of remarkable. I subsequently became very curious about kinesiology and was introduced to Dr. Versendahl's method, which is known as *contact reflex analysis*.
I became so intrigued I studied and mastered the principles of this technique.

According to Dr. Versendahl, the front of our hands are electrically positive and the backs of our hands are electrically negative. The tips of our fingers are neutral. The practitioner performs kinesiology testing by locating a body area with one hand and exerting pressure on the patient's outstretched (from the side) arm. If there is a problem with the tested area, the arm will go weak, like a short circuit. For example, when the neutral tip of the finger is held over the upper end of the sternum and the arm goes weak, it generally indicates that there is a heart muscle weakness. However, if you hold the negative, or reverse, side of the hand over the same area and the arm goes weak, it means that there is probably a B vitamin deficiency. Just above the breastbone is the notch of the lower neck. If you hold the tip of your finger, that is, neutral in this area and the arm goes weak, it reflects a thymus deficiency. If you hold the positive or negative part of your hand over that same area, it's a T-4 thyroid deficiency.

Kinesiology can help eliminate most mistakes associated with prescribing medications that patient's can't tolerate, are allergic to or simply don't need. The person holds the medication in his hand and runs his tongue over the roof of his mouth from back to front along the midline five to six times to improve the accuracy of the test. I have recently learned that putting your hand in a position like you are squeezing an orange and then rotating your hand over the navel area uncovers hidden problem areas. I also have patients tap the side of the hand next to the little finger 6 times. The practitioner then exerts pressure on the patients extended arm. If the arm gets weaker, it means that the medication probably will not agree with him. It could be he is allergic to it or the body just doesn't need it. I do not advocate the use of any supplement, homeopathic or medicinal, unless a patient has been tested by kinesiology. Some holistic practitioners believe that you have to hold the substance in your mouth before you test it. Others believe that you have to hold it up against your chest wall or your abdomen. I find that either approach provides acceptable results.

Kinesiology simplifies the practice of medicine. For example, a patient comes into the doctor's office with a sore throat. The physician examines the throat and sees that it is red. It is hard to differentiate whether the soreness is due to an infection, virus, strep, allergy or some other kind of bacteria. Sore throats are often misdiagnosed and treated incorrectly. Many doctors tend to treat most sore throats with an antibiotic. Often, it is the wrong antibiotic, or an antibiotic was not indicated. Some doctors do a throat culture, but it can be several days before the results are available. Either they have to wait for the results, treat the condition without them or rely on a rapid strep test that is fast, although not one-hundred percent accurate. Even if a throat culture is performed and the diagnosis confirmed, there are several antibiotics that could be effective against the bacteria. The doctor still does not know for certain which of the available antibiotics would be best for his patient. Kinesiology will help determine the correct medication to treat the problem.

Many times a patient will go to his physician with multiple symptoms. After a general physical examination, the doctor cannot find anything wrong. The physician can't formulate a treatment plan without an accurate diagnosis. Kinesiology eliminates this situation by pinpointing the problem even though it isn't identifiable in a regular exam or by laboratory work. Too many physicians treat the patient on the basis of laboratory results only. I believe that you treat the patient's symptoms and complaints with kinesiology test results *and* a physical exam and laboratory work. It continues to amaze me how many physicians do otherwise.

A very thorough physical can be done with kinesiology in less than a minute and a half. It will give you more information than an allopathic exam. Each of my patients gets a complete kinesiology exam even if they come in with a sore toe. I also listen to their heart and lungs and feel their stomach, and so forth. I find that many times patients will present a minor ailment and I will find something signifi-cant that has not been symptomatic enough to bring it to their attention. For example, a lady came in complaining of a sore knee. With a kinesiology examina-tion I discovered that her liver was abnormal. She finally admitted that she had an alcohol problem. Her knee problem was minor; therefore, we concentrated on treating her alcoholism and repairing her liver with supplements.

If the arm goes weak after a neutral test with the tip of the finger just below the left eye, you are likely to have a bacterial infection. You can put the tip of the finger to the navel; if the arm goes weak, you have a yeast infection. Place the tip of the finger about an inch or so below the umbilicus. If a weak arm is present, you have a virus infection. Holding the hand positive in a horizontal position in front of the eyes will indicate an allergy if the arm weakens. If a patient has a bacterial infection, antibiotics are indicated unless the patient requests alterna-tive therapy. In the case of a bacterial infection, I can determine whether it is staph or strep by placing the tips of the fingers just above the collarbone next to the neck. If the arm goes weak, strep is likely. Having made a definitive diagno-sis, I use kinesiology again to determine the proper treatment.

First, I select a substance that I feel will work and have them hold it. If the arm stays strong, I know it will agree with them. Then I have them hold the medi-cine and I touch the bacterial point, and if it's the right antibiotic, the arm will remain strong. Again, if it's staph or strep, you'll want to test it against that point also.

My two rules are:

- Don't give anything unless the person holding it remains with a strong arm.

- It has to correct the weak reflex. By correcting, I mean changing from a weak reflex to a strong reflex.

Your body will tell you the correct dosage in addition to the proper supplement if it is properly asked. If a person holds a bottle of vitamin C in his hand and his arm weakens, he probably doesn't tolerate or need that particular vitamin. This suggests the following:

- Try another brand and the arm will stay strong, indicating that there is a difference in the composition of the vitamin C from one company to another.

This is very common, especially with vitamin E. There is a d-alpha vitamin E that is natural, and there is a dl-alpha tocopherol vitamin E that is synthetic. Many people not knowing the difference buy the synthetic vitamin E because it is cheaper. Most people do not test well for a synthetic. A lot of the side effects attributed to vitamin E are the result of a synthetic dose. Bargains like synthetic vitamin E may help your pocketbook in the short term but will harm your health in the long term.

Serious illnesses such as cancer and heart disease oftentimes do not exhibit early symptoms. Kinesiology provides the physician with an opportunity to address the problem before the patient is symptomatic.

Jean, a sister of a good friend, had suffered from abdominal pain for several months, causing her to spend considerable amounts of time bedridden. Her brother explained to me that she had been evaluated and treated with great expense at a well-known clinic without any improvement. He asked me to see her. I examined her abdomen with kinesiology. It took only several minutes to determine that the abdominal pain was due to a pinched nerve in her back. I recommended that she see a chiropractor, and within a short time she was pain-free.

In another case, an elderly gentleman was hospitalized at the same clinic with a serious leg infection. Regardless of the increased doses of antibiotics, the infection was worsening. The patient discharged himself from the hospital in frustration and came to see me as a new patient. With the aid of kinesiology I diagnosed a yeast infection (which is made worse with antibiotics) and treated him with a nutritional program. He called two weeks later to say that his infection had cleared and he was back playing golf. I saw him only once.

A middle-aged husband and father was diagnosed at the same clinic with excess fluid in the pericardial sac surrounding the heart. Numerous expensive studies were performed without finding the cause of the effusion. He was told that with enough testing the cause would eventually be found. In an attempt to avoid the extra testing and expense, he came to see me as a new patient. It was easy to pinpoint the cause of the effusion as a parasite infection. I prescribed an herbal combination and he proceeded to get better. When he returned to the original medical facility, he was laughed at when he told his physicians that he was being treated for parasites. Undaunted, he continued his parasite treatment program and the effusion was resolved.

I want to make it clear that by using these cases as examples, I am not knocking this specific clinic. They have had an excellent reputation for a long time. I have been treated by them myself. I am using these cases only as an example that at the very best medical institutions there is a need for different thinking and for the use of alternative medicine.

A layperson can learn to perform kinesiology testing by doing the following:

- Face the subject.

- Apply downward pressure to their wrist with their arm extended, palm down, before testing to determine their strength.

- To see if they are testable, point your finger at the bridge of their nose between the eyes. If they are testable, their arm will become weak.

- Before testing it is always wise to make their testing more accurate by:

  ➤ running their tongue over the roof of their mouth back to front at least six times,

  ➤ tap the side of either hand by the little finger six times,

  ➤ rotate your flexed hand right and left over their umbilicus.

- For testing medication, have them hold the substance in either hand. If the arm shows signs of weakness, they should not take it. If they test strong, you can determine the number of pills per day by asking them to think about a day's dose and then place one, two, three, four, and so forth, into their hand to see the amount they are strong on. They should be weak on all doses except the one best tolerated. Remember, practice makes perfect.

My fondest wish is to have all physicians learn kinesiology. Prior to acquiring this skill, I had seven to fifteen patients in the hospital on any given day. Now I admit less than three patients in a year. What could be more cost-effective? Also, it would give physicians another diagnostic tool and permit them to more accurately prescribe medications. As noted in the April 1998 issue of the *Journal of the American Medical Association,* there were over 100,000 deaths from drugs that were prescribed and/or used *properly.*

Chiropractic

While I was in medical school, my father injured his back. He'd always gone to chiropractors for his back pain, yet while working toward my medical degree, I'd been taught chiropractic was without value. I implored my father to see an orthopedic surgeon and, consequently, Dad was hospitalized and put into pelvic traction for one week. He did not appreciate this remedy in the least. I prevailed upon him to keep trying it, as this was the right treatment. After the first week, my father showed no signs of improvement, so he signed himself out of the hospital and went to see his chiropractor. With one manipulation he was fine, and the total cost was four dollars. I'm not sure of a week's hospital cost but it was more than he liked. Since it didn't help him, it was more than necessary to leave there and seek successful treatment elsewhere.

I'd never given much thought to chiropractic until a number of years later when I was having considerable trouble with my right knee, ankle and foot. I was getting fluid on the knee and my toes were painfully swollen, so I went to a number of different well-recognized medical authorities to find the cause and cure. Among them was Dr. McGuire, the team physician of the Green Bay Packers. I also went to Cleveland Clinic, the University of Michigan, the University of Arizona and several local physicians.

All of them did their best; however, nothing helped my problems. Consequently, I was on and off crutches for several years. Trying to deliver babies and perform general surgery while leaning on crutches was, should I say, difficult. I couldn't find relief, except for an anti-inflammatory drug no longer available on the market. No number of pain pills seemed to help. When trying to hunt or walk in the woods, each step would cause me to cry in pain. I became very discouraged and disillusioned with the medical treatment for my problem.

I traveled to Dallas for a holistic medical convention, arriving on crutches. My medical practice partner was organizing the convention. He asked his brother, Ray Massner, D.C., to adjust my back, and though I was still skeptical about chiropractic medicine, I decided I had nothing to lose. The morning after Dr. Massner adjusted my back, I still wasn't much better. An herbalist offered to mix up a preparation to help my back and I willingly obliged. The following day I felt so much better that I returned home to Michigan carrying my crutches!

Six to eight weeks later, my painful back and leg symptoms returned. I immediately called the herbalist for another dose of his elixir but unfortunately it didn't work this time. After evaluating the situation, I decided that it might have been the chiropractic manipulation that was effective. Subsequent chiropractic manipulation successfully resolved my symptoms caused by a subluxation between my fourth and fifth lumbar vertebrae. Over twenty years later, I have yet to talk to any physician who believes that manipulation would eliminate the fluid on my knee.

I eventually transferred my practice from Michigan to Prescott, Arizona, where I worked in partnership with Dr. Massner for nine years. During this period I saw astounding results with chiropractic. Dr. Massner healed patients who would otherwise have been left in considerable pain or with other symptoms. I believe that chiropractic works, but not in all cases. I regularly recommend chiropractic to those patients that I feel have a correctable subluxation. My objection to chiropractic medicine is that many practitioners over-treat. Too many adjustments are provided over too long a period of time. If the adjustments don't result in a marked improvement in a patient's symptoms in a matter of three to six weeks, they should either stop the adjustments or seek another chiropractor.

As with the case of my father, chiropractic treatment of other family members stands out vividly in my mind. My six-year-old granddaughter had been very ill with a high temperature, sore throat and cough, for which I prescribed an antibiotic. Five days later she coughed up some blood. I thought I had missed diagnosing pneumonia. After Dr. Massner took a chest x-ray and found it clear, I re-examined her and was about to return home with her when he asked if he could examine my granddaughter, though I doubted there was anything he could do for her. She had been lying around the house, not playing with her friends and not eating for some time. I couldn't conceive of how chiropractic could help her, yet I consented because I didn't believe chiropractic could harm her. He worked on her ten minutes, I took her home, and within thirty minutes she was back to her old self. The cough subsided and the chronic stomach pain was gone. She went outside and started playing with her friends, her energy level markedly increased. I still have trouble believing it, even though a number of years ago have gone by and, to my knowledge; she has not had stomach problems since.

A month after the experience with my granddaughter, my son-in-law came to visit. He arrived with significant back pain. I decided that his back problem was due to his three-hundred-plus pounds of body weight. He'd also broken his ankle two years earlier and metal bars were inserted into his ankle, resulting in a painful limp. After a year and a great deal of pain, the metal bars were removed but he was still experiencing considerable pain. I came to the conclusion that chiropractic could be beneficial, so I asked Dr. Massner to treat him, suggesting that part of his problem was due to the old ankle fracture.

When Dr. Massner said, "Well, let's fix the ankle," I didn't anticipate this approach. Dr. Massner reduced the ankle, which had apparently been subluxed, and again within thirty minutes the pain was gone. You can imagine how upset my son-in-law was when he realized he'd been in pain for two years and that all he needed was a simple ankle adjustment. Two remarkable cases in my first six months of being associated with Dr. Massner opened my eyes to the possibilities of chiropractic.

There is a special technique of chiropractic called *cranial manipulation*. A young girl had been born deaf and was brought to Dr. Massner for help when all else failed to produce even a slight amount of hearing. After a number of cranial adjustments, her hearing miraculously returned and she was hearing sounds for the first time. I read a letter she had written to Dr. Massner and one line still stands out in my memory: "My hearing is so good now that I can hear a drop of rain fall on a blade of grass." I'll never forget her joy.

I have been without crutches and able to climb the mountains around Prescott. I have, though, experienced several exacerbations of my back problems, both involving disc disease. My back pain was resolved to the point that I could return to work within one week by using a combination of acupuncture, chiro-practic and massage, and was essentially pain-free within two weeks. Do I believe in chiropractic? You bet! And you should too, *for selective cases.* Sometimes joints and vertebrae get out of position and many times they'll re-align on their own. But when they don't, think about a chiropractic adjustment. Other methods of resolving joint malposition include certain types of massage, myofacial release and rolfing. I oftentimes refer patients to specialists trained in these techniques, with good results.

I've learned several chiropractic techniques such as adjusting the dorsal spine, adjusting the first and second cervical vertebrae and adjusting ankles, shoulders and elbows. However, I do very few manipulative procedures and usually refer my patients to a chiropractor. Even though I don't do many manipulations, there have been two occasions where it was helpful and probably should have been considered by the attending physician. Both cases involved radicular pain which is a condition wherein the dorsal spine gets out of alignment and pinches one of the nerves, thus causing considerable pain.

In the first case, a patient of mine was seen in the emergency room due to an experience with severe chest pain. X-rays, blood work and an electrocardiogram were performed. The emergency room physician had become frustrated trying to determine the origin of the pain. At one a.m., he asked me to see the patient. After reviewing her chart I checked her back and found it to be out of alignment. With a simple adjustment, her chest pain was gone.

An orderly at the hospital was complaining of right-upper abdominal pain. The attending physician ordered gastrointestinal x-rays, gall bladder x-rays, an ultrasound of the gallbladder and blood tests. All his test results were normal; however, the orderly still had pain. He asked me what I thought could be causing his pain. With a brief exam I found a pinched nerve in his back and adjusted him. The pain ceased. Radicular pain caused by a pinched nerve is very common and may cause pelvic and abdominal pain as well as chest pain. All too often radicular pain is not considered in the differential diagnosis. Unfortunately, this "blindness" is due to a lack of chiropractic training in our studies.

In the earlier section on kinesiology, I related the case of Jean, who had been bedridden for several months with abdominal pain also due to a pinched nerve in her back.

Homeopathy

Homeopathy is the antithesis of allopathic medicine. Allopathic medicine uses large doses of chemicals. The larger the dose, the more potent the medication and, correspondingly, the more the side effects. With homeopathy, the smaller the dose the more potent it is. Very few homeopathic medications have significant side effects.

There is a documented similarity between the toxicological action of a substance and its therapeutic action. In Hippocrates' time, white hellebore produced cholera-like diarrhea when taken in large doses. A homeopathic preparation was successfully used to treat cholera. Cantharis tincture in toxic doses causes bladder inflammation and blood in the urine. When taken in infinitesimal doses, it is effective treatment for the same illnesses.

Hippocrates believed that the things that cause a disease could also cure it. It was not until the end of the eighteenth century that German physician, Dr. S. Hahnemann, observed that cinchona, a remedy used to treat certain types of malaria fever, caused a fever similar to malaria when taken in large doses. Dr. Hahnemann tested various herbal combinations on both himself and his students. He proved that the resulting symptoms caused by toxic doses of various herbs and minerals such as aconite, belladonna, and ipecac, could be treated by infinitesimal doses of the same substances.

Homeopathic principles were studied throughout the 1800s. In early 1900, there were a number of homeopathic medical schools throughout the United States. Allopathic schools and infighting among various homeopathic practitioners drove them out of existence. Today, homeopathy is regaining acceptance in the United States. It is even being taught in some of our major medical schools. In Great Britain the Queen has her own homeopathic physician. Homeopathy is also widely practiced in Europe and India.

Treating the patient with homeopathy requires a very detailed history, a clear description of the symptoms and an evaluation of the patient's general behavior. General behavior includes likes and dislikes in food and sexual behaviors, as well as dream and sleep disorders. The variety of treatment regimens and their requirements must be matched specifically to functional symptoms, making the practice of homeopathy more difficult than allopathic medicine.

Dr. Hahnemann developed homeopathy and is credited with the emergence of this type of medicine. He disagreed with some of the allopathic treatments of the time just, as I do with some current regimens. Thankfully, many of the questionable allopathic treatments at that time, such as bloodletting and not using aseptic techniques, and so on, have been discarded. Another common practice, the removal of the tonsils and adenoids, is no longer the standard. I remember bringing in four or five children from one family and doing tonsillectomies on all of them. We finally realized it was not good medicine. Tonsillectomies and adenoidectomies are now restricted to patients with repeated infections of the tonsils or recurrent ear infections.

Subtotal hysterectomy, a common procedure in the early years of my practice, is no longer routinely performed. A number of thyroid tests have been discarded in favor of newer, more reliable testing. Medicine is evolving and progressing. It must utilize the established treatment regimens while exploring new horizons. Doctors have to be open-minded and willing to accept changes for the betterment of their patients.

Homeopathy is a therapeutic method based on the Law of Similars, which says that like corrects like. Homeopathy employs medicinal substances of many different plants and animals in weak or infinitesimal doses. Hippocrates first observed this principle over twenty-five centuries ago; however, it was Dr. Hahnemann who eventually brought this school of medicine to prominence. Homeopathy works by stimulating the defense mechanisms of the body to make it work more effectively, so only small doses of homeopathic medicine are needed. Allopathic chemical drugs work in opposition to the body's mechanism. Consequently, stronger allopathic medications are needed to affect the symptoms. These mega doses of allopathic drugs cause many side effects.

A patient recently brought in a cartoon showing a pharmacist dispensing medication to a patient. The caption read: "This bottle is your prescription. These other five bottles are to take care of the side effects." I think this sums up what is happening with many of our medicinal therapies today. Gross reactions between different drugs are widespread. In Phoenix, a woman recently died because of a reaction between her antihistamine and her antibiotic.

There are over 2,800 homeopathic remedies. These elements are mixed with an alcohol solution and are then serially diluted. With each dilution they are shaken, secussed, and then diluted again until a very diluted solution is obtained. The different dilutions are then identified by means of an "X" or a "C," with the higher the number the more the dilution. 6X is not as diluted as a 12X or a 30X or a 200X. Most of the elements are so diluted that if you analyzed them you would not find one single molecule of the original substance. What remains in the solution is the "energy" of the original element.

Until I went into partnership with Dr. Massner, I didn't know anything about homeopathy. Consequently, the theory was hard for me to accept. I'd earned a degree in chemistry before entering medical school and homeopathy was dramatically opposed to what I had been taught. However, I believe it is important for a physician to keep an open mind and investigate anything that might enable him to help his patients. After observing his results, I became intrigued and subsequently took courses in homeopathy. I received my Arizona Medical License in homeopathic medicine in April in 1993.

There are two types of homeopathy practiced today. I was taught the classical form of homeopathy. Classical homeopaths treat with a single remedy zeroing in like a rifle shot on a target. Non-classical homeopaths use a shotgun approach. They utilize a number of different remedies mixed together to score a hit. The latter approach is far simpler but much less specific. In an effort to balance economy with effectiveness, there have been a number of these shotgun preparations sold at health food store counters to patients who are treating themselves.

Many people try to discredit homeopathy by saying it's simply a placebo. I disagree for several reasons. There have been a number of experiments performed on animals with good clinical results. These animals couldn't differentiate between medicine and a placebo; also, I've had several cases early in my homeo-pathic experience proving its effectiveness.

In the first case, an elderly woman came in with arthritis. I treated her with Rhus Tox, a dilution of poison ivy. In the particular strength I gave her, there was no possibility that any molecules of the original poison ivy remained in the remedy. Notwithstanding, the patient developed a very severe case of poison ivy. The symptoms of the poison ivy persisted for six weeks in spite of my efforts to neutralize it and create an antidote. The rash ultimately cleared. We noted an improvement in her arthritic symptoms and amazingly large benign lesions also cleared up. The results proved the effectiveness of the remedy and showed me that without a molecule of the substance being present, the energy factor could simulate a disease.

A gentleman in his mid-twenties came into the office with a sinus infection. This was one of the most severe sinus infections I've seen in my entire practice. I explained the seriousness of his condition and the possibility of it leading to meningitis. Through kinesiology I selected one of the most potent oral antibi-otics available in hope that he could avoid hospitalization. He asked about the cost of the antibiotic and I told him it would be over $100. He told me he couldn't afford that and needed something less expensive. He asked if there was anything less costly, but still effective. I suggested a $7 homeopathic remedy. He agreed to try it first.

After administering the homeopathic remedy I instructed him to get the expensive prescription filled in case he should get worse over the weekend. Regardless, I wanted to hear from him on Monday regarding his progress. I did not anticipate any significant improvement in his symptoms for at least a week. A ten-to-fourteen day treatment regimen was likely. I suspected any antibiotic treatment would stop the infection's progress before providing improvement. When he called on Monday I was amazed to hear that he was without symptoms and greatly improved. Another success story for an inexpensive homeopathic treatment!

Let me give you an idea of the remedies for several different symptoms:

I had mentioned Rhus Toxicodendrom, commonly known as poison ivy. The symptoms caused by this plant are well known to most. On the skin it causes swelling and vesicular eruptions. Unknown to most people, it can also cause painful stiffness of tendons and connective tissue, which is relieved by motion. It also affects the nervous system and can cause depression. These characteristic symptoms can be improved by motion or by changing position, by heat and hot compresses and can become better during hot and dry weather. However, these symptoms are aggravated by humidity, wet, cold atmospheric changes and contact with moist objects. The symptoms worsen when a person begins to move or is extremely tired. Although they get worse when the patient begins to move, they improve after additional motion. The specific modality of sensation is stiffness and bruising pain and feeling as if cold water were being poured over the body. The mucous symptoms can be hoarseness when the patient begins to speak or sing, dryness of the mouth and intense thirst for cold water or milk. Rhus Tox can be used for any of the aforementioned symptoms as well as for sprains, dislocations, muscular fatigue and any rheumatism aggravated by an increase in humidity.

Kali Bichromiuim is a potassium dichromate salt especially useful in cases of mucosal inflammation with large amounts of thick, yellow or green sticky secretion. The symptoms are aggravated by exposure to cold, and improve with heat. It was the remedy that I used on the patient with the severe sinusitis. Kali Bichromium is also used to treat aphis ulcers, gastric pain and burning stomach ulcers, nausea, and gas following meals, diarrhea associated with arthritis symptoms, left sciatica and pain in the soles of the feet especially in the heels.

There are numerous excellent books on homeopathy. There are also courses in homeopathy for the physician and also for the layman. Some courses are very extensive and take several years to complete. Anyone interested in becoming a homeopath should consider attending the classes taught by Vega Rosenberg in Flagstaff, Arizona. I consider him to be one of the brightest minds in the field of homeopathic education.

Chelation Therapy

Chelation means to grasp, or claw. In a medical application, chelating agents grasp or bind metastatic or pathological mineral deposits in our body, enabling us to excrete them. Chelation was first used in 1941 to treat lead poisoning. A great number of physicians have used it extensively since the 1960s. Thousands of articles related to its use have been published. It is not approved by the AMA and is not recommended by most doctors. There are two major reasons chelation is not more widely used. Most physicians have deferred an educated opinion to that of the AMA and secondly, chelation works and thereby negates the need for expensive surgical procedures. I am a proponent of chelation therapy because it treats the problems and doesn't simply mask the symptoms or set aside the problem temporarily. It is a very good treatment for some heavy metal toxic conditions such as lead poisoning.

I began performing intravenous chelation therapy through the prompting of my friend, Dave Bennett. Dave sustained a myocardial infarction and was bound and determined to be treated with chelation therapy and prodded me until I learned how to administer intravenous chelation therapy. It has been over 20 years and he is still doing fine. As it is normally practiced in the United States, intravenous chelation therapy is administered with an IV drip of EDTA (Ethelene-diaminotetra acetic acid.) It is often mixed with other substances such as lidocaine, heparin, magnesium, B vitamins and vitamin C. Other doctors use their own choice of drug combinations. I add an oral multiple vitamin supplement to the above program and vary the dose for each individual.

The book *By-passing the By-pass*, discusses chelation therapy in detail and recommends its use to avoid having heart bypass surgery. I have been using chelation therapy for over twenty years and find it has helped patients in over eighty percent of the cases. I usually reserve its use for circulatory problems such as intermittent claudicating or atheriosclerotic heart disease, sometimes referred to as coronary heart disease. For patients with angina, the effects are quite obvious. Any disease process affected by poor circulation can often be improved by chelation. It has been used for other conditions such as heavy metal toxicity, arthritis, porphyria, scleroderma and hypertension. It is a very good treatment for non-hemmoraghic stroke, if not the best I have found. Vitamin A and mineral depletion can be a side effect, usually requiring supplementation. There are over twenty biochemical reactions attributed to chelating action. However, I am certain there are many more positive effects yet to be investigated. One of the most significant to date is its ability to affect nitrous oxide (NO).

Oral chelating agents in the form of a vitamin-mineral-herbal supplement can also be used to improve the circulation. Chelation works on all the blood vessels in your body. Oral chelation is comparatively inexpensive and quite effective. The exact dosage of medication is best determined by kinesiology. Every person is different and your uniqueness changes. One month your body may need one thing and three months later the requirements will change. Red blood cells constantly replace old ones every 120 days. Your surface stomach and gastrointestinal cells are replaced every five to seven days. Most other cells in your body are replaced at different rates but usually within ninety days. After a year has passed, except for brain cells, you're almost an entirely different cellular individual. The idea behind chelation and the use of proper thinking and nutrition is to nourish and repair each new cell as they are made. Hopefully, the new cells will be better than those they replace.

A specialist in Marquette, Michigan, diagnosed a patient with Alzheimer's disease. The gentleman needed to be placed in a nursing home. No beds were available, so he was transferred to our hospital to await placement. I thought as long as the patient was in our hospital waiting for a bed, I would do more than merely provide nursing care. After five chelation treatments he was up and about, fully coherent, and I was able to confidently discharge him back to his home. If it had not been for the chelation he would have likely spent his remaining days in a nursing facility. Obviously a wrong diagnosis had been made.

A second case involved the eighty-four year-old father of a very close friend. The father sustained a complete stroke and was paralyzed on the complete left side of his body. He was hospitalized one-hundred miles away from his home. He had been there for seven days when the son was told that his father should be placed in a nursing home. I suggested to my friend that he transfer his father to our hospital. After his transfer to our facility, I elected to use a regimen of chelation therapy, noting an improvement after several treatments. I called the physiotherapy department of a rehabilitation hospital to place this patient in the stroke rehab unit, but no beds were available. While awaiting transfer, I gave him a total of eighteen chelation treatments.

Guess what? He walked out of the hospital after the eighteenth treatment without assistance and went home without a nurse or caregiver. A week later the stroke unit called to say they had a bed available. I informed them he already had a bed and it was in his own home. He lived to be ninety-two years old, and I believe he had chelation therapy to thank for those extra years.

In the past six months I have had two patients who were presented in wheel chairs and on oxygen. One was seventy-five and the other was eighty-three. Both had been told by the V.A. Hospital that they were not surgical candidates and were given only a few months to live (see testimonials.) After ten chelations they were markedly improved and after approximately thirty treatments, they were symptom-free, up and about, out of wheel chairs and off oxygen. The eighty-three year-old was back to teaching dance classes at one of our local colleges. The seventy-five year-old was back home living alone and fishing to his heart's content.

The past six months have also re-convinced me of chelation's positive effects not only in coronary heart disease with angina but also in congestive heart failure, peripheral vascular disease with leg pain when walking and the improvement in persons suffering from cerebral vascular insufficiency.

Chelation is a viable option for anyone considering surgical treatment for vascular problems. I find it to be safer than aspirin if treatment guidelines are followed. The treatments usually cost about $100, certainly far less expensive than vascular surgery. I believe it is medical malpractice for a doctor not to give this option to a patient.

Most EDTA therapies require approximately twenty to thirty treatments. It is recommended that a patient receive five to ten chelation treatments a year thereafter, once the problem is controlled. A patient also needs to continue a regular exercise program and follow his prescribed diet. The diet should be individually designed, as each person often needs a specific diet depending on their weight, cholesterol and triglyceride levels, their sugar tolerance, age, and all other medical factors. If a patient takes oral chelation during and/or after intravenous chelation, the necessity of taking further yearly intravenous chelation treatments can often be avoided.

I have been told that in Australia a patient has to have a trial of chelation therapy *before* he can be a candidate for surgery.

It has been found to be of benefit in a number of diseases. A partial list includes:

- angina pectoris
- coronary artery disease
- scleroderma
- multiple sclerosis
- digitalis intoxication
- arteriosclerosis
- diabetic gangrene
- kidney stones
- lead poisoning
- excessive iron deposits
- senility
- liver function

Recently, oral chelation with EDTA has been advocated. I tried it on my mother thirty years ago. She laughed and said she didn't know if it helped her arteries but it sure was a good laxative!

Magnesium–EDTA is the chemical that is used in intravenous therapy that takes approximately three hours to administer. Now they are recommending calcium-EDTA intravenously. It can be given over a ten-minute period of time rather than three hours. It has the advantage that it does not cause vein irritation and obviously costs less. We charge $30.00 for this treatment and I am now recommending it. World-renowned expert on chelation therapy, Gary Gordon, also recommends this *Fast Push* form of chelation.

EDTA is many times safer than aspirin. Coronary artery bypass (CAB) surgery is very expensive and according to the *New England Journal of Medicine*, when compared to less risky and less invasive medical therapy, appears neither to prolong life nor to prevent myocardial infarction in patients with mild angina or who are asymptomatic after heart attack in the five-year period after coronary angiography.

The AMA recognizes chelation therapy as a treatment for heavy metal poisoning such as lead, aluminum, and cadmium.

But neither the FDA nor the AMA admits that chelation appears to be one of the most powerful, safest and least-expensive treatments for heart disease that we have now available.

Multiple studies and millions of patient attest to the wonderful benefits of chelation therapy—I among them! (Read "Stroke of Luck," a later chapter.)

Aromatherapy

Aromatherapy is back! Its popularity is gaining it wide use and acceptance. It is a very old form of medicinal therapy and has been practiced for thousands of years. The Egyptians used oils for religious as well as for healing purposes. We know from the Bible that much importance was attributed to oils. Frankincense and myrrh were brought as tribute to the Christ child. The Wise Men would not have done this if oils were not considered a precious gift. Biblical references mention the use of frankincense, sandalwood and patchouli oils. Scripture also recommends hyssop, myrrh and cinnamon for treatment of infectious diseases.

There are many aroma oils used for treating medical and emotional symptoms. A friend of mine, Terry Shephard Friedman, M.D., has used them extensively

and has recently written an excellent book, *Freedom Through Health*.
Dr. Friedman's book discusses his ideas on holistic medicine and includes a chapter on aromatic oils and their applications. These oils are distilled from plants. Many oils are of inferior quality because they are not distilled at the right temperature and/or extracted with various chemicals or overly diluted. This detracts from the oil's effectiveness.

The aromatic oils I use in my practice are supplied by Young's Living Oils and I believe they are the best available. Using anything less might cause side effects such as skin rashes or produce less than desired results. These oils can alleviate a wide variety of symptoms including emotional distress, infectious disease and allergic reactions. They've also been beneficial in the treatment of arthritis, asthma, back pain and parasite infections.

The first time I used aromatherapy, a lady came into the office with an acute asthmatic attack brought on by her exposure to molds. She had a history of environmental illnesses with extreme sensitivity. Her asthma symptoms were very severe. I debated giving her intravenous steroids, adrenaline, and so forth, when something told me to try aromatherapy first. I have a kit of approximately sixty various aromatic oils and oil blends in my office. I did some intuitive kinesiology on her and selected eucalyptus. I applied a drop of eucalyptus to the inner aspects of each wrist, a little under her nose and some on both lung points, just immediately below the mid-portion of both collarbones. Much to her surprise, and mine, her asthma was one-hundred percent reversed in two minutes. She was breathing fine with no symptoms. One dose was sufficient. I saw her later in the week. She was free of any symptoms. The patient will readily attest to its effectiveness.

Another patient was having extreme difficulty due to sensitivity to cigarette smoke. When I saw her she was coughing and had labored breathing. I did intuitive kinesiology and arrived at an oil blend called RC. It is a mixture of various aromatic oils. I applied them to the same areas as with the first patient. Within ten minutes she was entirely free of any symptoms.

A third patient came to the office and appeared to have been drinking excessively. She was incoherent, dizzy, and feeling somewhat nauseated. Her history revealed that she had recently undergone dental work and apparently had been given an anesthetic that did not agree with her. These symptoms occurred shortly following the anesthetic and persisted for almost two days. Since the symptoms were not improving, the patient came in for evaluation and treatment. I knew of no allopathic therapy that would help her in this situation.

I elected to try aromatherapy. Within fifteen to twenty minutes, using one application of the oil rubbed on her skin, her symptoms were resolved. The following week, she told me that her symptoms had not returned.

I once experienced a severe burning sensation from an insect bite. I applied lavender oil to the bite and within a minute the burning sensation was alleviated. Lavender can be effective treatment for a number of different conditions. It has been used therapeutically for attention deficit disorder and for burns. It also acts as an above-average antihistamine and is therefore excellent for allergy therapy.

Hyperactivity, insomnia, stretch marks, sunburn, anger, apathy, bitterness, correction of bad habits, treating resentment, tension and general wellbeing have been positively affected by lavender. There are no allopathic drugs that can produce all these positive benefits without side effects.

In my opinion, aromatic oil will be used more frequently in the future. One area of interest will be in the treatment of infections. Bacteria are becoming resistant to known antibiotics and viruses are developing immunity to our current antibiotics. Most of you do not remember the 1918 influenza epidemic that killed over twenty million people. Most people in the world today have lower, weaker immune systems due to pollution, increased stress and poorer eating habits. Aroma oils have been found to be very effective in fighting a number of these antibiotic-resistant illnesses, including the plague.

In the recent past, there has been a large increase in deaths from infectious diseases worldwide. We are noting a resurgence of tuberculosis, which is drug-resistant. In the immediate future there will be more deaths from infectious disease due to viruses. Some aromatic oils, which have shown antiviral and antibacterial properties, are lemon oil, lavender, hyssop, frankincense, peppermint, clove, thyme and others. According to Dr. Friedman's research, frankincense, myrrh and sage have been found to be effective against some cancers. Germanium can help diabetics, and Yang Yang is beneficial in the control of cardiac arrhythmia. Clary sage is a natural estrogen precursor.

For the sake of you and your loved ones, I strongly suggest that you become familiar with aromatic oils and their benefits and side effects.

Nutritional Therapy

Nutritional therapy is perhaps the most beneficial area of alternative medicine. While in the Air Force, I had a number of patients return from Europe with vitamin and other supplements. Being a good allopathic physician, I told them these substances wouldn't do them any good and often advised them to stop. After all, it was only six years since I had graduated from the University of Michigan. "If I hadn't been taught it, it probably wasn't any good."

After my discharge, a friend introduced me to Standard Process products and nutritional therapy. He told me of all the different illnesses that could be cured or improved using natural, non-synthetic nutritional therapy. I found the concept very hard to accept. However, keeping an open mind I agreed to some clinical trials. It was an endocardiogram that convinced me that nutritional therapy was an effective modality. The endocardiogram was used on a patient with a cardiac arrhythmia. After reviewing the recording, my friend administered a pure vitamin B in chewable form. After chewing the tablet for two minutes the endocardiogram returned to normal. Visible proof, on this one occasion, that nutrition worked.

I continued to research nutritional therapy and found that other conditions could be treated with this method. A vitamin E extract called Cataplex E-2 works as well as or better than nitroglycerin for angina. Unlike nitroglycerin, it can be used in large amounts without any side effects.

Nutrition also plays a big role in cancer therapy. I was associated for a year with the Gerson Cancer Clinic in Sedona, Arizona. Nutritional therapy was the mainstay of the therapy. The Gerson therapy has been around for forty or fifty years, producing good results in the treatment of many different forms of cancer and degenerative problems. The treatment included freshly squeezed juices, organic vegetables, low-protein and low-salt diets. Gerson employed other nutritional modalities along with the diet, such as thyroid, potassium and pancreas extract. Hydrochloric acid was added to help digest food, and coffee enemas were administered to detoxify the colon.

There are nutritional products for diabetes, hypoglycemia, arthritis and a variety of digestive disorders. There are also nutritional therapies to correct or alleviate symptoms for which there is no allopathic treatment. I have progressively administered more and more nutritional therapies rather than drug therapies to avoid side effects and reduce the patient's expenses.

Recently science discovered that dendrites in the brain could actually be stimulated to regrow through nutritional therapy. Granted, the dendrites do not regrow to their original form and level of action, but patients with some forms of early Alzheimer's and brain damage induced by alcohol, and so forth, could actually be improved through the use of nutritional supplements. Preliminary studies have shown even neurons can be regrown.

A good friend developed cancer of the pancreas in his late twenties. He was treated with nutritional supplements to eradicate parasites prior to his surgery. It has been over nine years and he has no sign of cancer, and the Mayo Clinic surgeons can't understand it. Again, I attribute his survival to immune enhancement and parasite reduction through nutrition.

Thousands, of books and articles have been written on various aspects of nutrition. If you are motivated, you can find information on almost any subject. Some general observations I have regarding nutritional therapy might prove helpful to you. The human body needs food, water and oxygen. Our body can manufacture many substances; however, those that the body doesn't synthesize must be ingested. Like building a house, the better the material, the longer the house will last. Unfortunately, we can't get the best food and water today. Our soils have been depleted of minerals, an essential part of our basic building blocks.

Farmers have tried to increase their yield by using chemical fertilizers and chemical sprays to kill insects. Unfortunately, they reject the idea that insects don't usually bother healthy plants, but only those sick and/or deficient in minerals. Similarly, if we keep our bodies well nourished our immune systems will prevent us from getting sick. Isn't it better to prevent illness than to disobey the laws of nature and have to treat an illness? I believe we need to emphasize wellness rather than illness. In the Orient, doctors are paid to keep a patient well. They are not paid to treat illness!

All of us need supplementation of specific vitamins, minerals, amino acids, antioxidants, enzymes, and so forth, because of poor dietary habits or because of inferior food products. In general, nonorganic food is so adulterated that our digestive system must work overtime. The toxins contained in our food put a burden on our immune system. Thus, we are more susceptible to illness. Even organic food is often mineral-deficient. Too many of us live in polluted areas, putting another great strain on the immune system. Getting the proper nutritional supplementation will help to overcome the deficiencies and excesses in our diets.

Unfortunately many health-food store supplements are not as good as claimed. They are sold more for profit than to improve a person's health. The best available method of determining what is good for you is kinesiology testing.

Another area of concern is the nutritional status of children. More and more examples of violent behavior involving children are reported each day. The media is quick to incriminate guns, poor parental supervision and violence on television, and so on. I'm sure that all of these play a role, but I believe the main cause of this antisocial behavior is specific vitamin, mineral, and amino acid deficiencies. *Our children are not eating correctly!* The most common nutritional deficiencies found in children are B vitamins, zinc and magnesium, the trace mineral lithium and the amino acids L-phenylalanine, glutamine and tyrosine. These deficiencies are common in children with learning disabilities, hyperactivity, attention deficit disorder (ADD), anger and difficulties with self-control.

Teach your children well and *early* the following basic nutritional facts:

- Digestion requires more energy than any other function.

- Your body can only digest one concentrated food at a time. Any food other than fruits and vegetables is concentrated.

- The enzymes renin and lactase are usually gone by age three. Therefore adults don't tolerate milk as well because it contains casein, which forms hard-to-digest curds and thus requires more energy to digest.

- Heat destroys enzymes and amino acids. It is more nutritious to eat raw or lightly cooked (steamed) foods.

- Fruits have the highest water content and essential nutrients of any food.

- Fruits should beaten raw rather than cooked.

- Don't drink while eating. It dilutes your stomach acid, which decreases your food digestion and assimilation.

- Sugar is empty calories. Excess fat and cholesterol cause your body to want to eat more to obtain your needed nutrients. This causes increased insulin productions that can cause hypoglycemia, and often insulin resistance that leads to diabetes.

- Soda pop contains phosphoric acid, malic acid and carbonic acid, which are bad for your teeth and upset the pH balance of your body.

- Avoid processed food as much as possible, especially simple carbohydrates.

Hydrogen Peroxide Therapy

Hydrogen peroxide (H_2O_2) is found naturally in fresh fruits, vegetables, rain, snow and in the first secretion of mother's milk. Also, the body produces very small amounts of hydrogen peroxide as part of the immune system defenses. The Food and Drug Administration has approved hydrogen peroxide for use as a food preservative and a topical antiseptic solution. It has not been approved for intravenous use, although its value has been documented in 7,000 medical journal articles since 1920.

In addition to viral infections and emphysema, it has been beneficial in the treatment of immune dysfunction and tissue hypoxia (low oxygen content.) H_2O_2 has also been found to increase the effectiveness of radiation therapy. The following conditions can be improved to varying degrees with intravenous hydrogen peroxide:

- Poor circulation
- Stroke and memory
- Heart disease
- Angina
- Gangrene
- Vascular headaches
- Raynaud's
- Asthma
- Chronic bronchitis
- Emphysema
- Influenza
- Shingles
- Cold sores
- Systemic chronic Candida
- Chronic fatigue syndrome

- AIDS

- Parasites

- Acute and chronic viral infections

- Multiple Sclerosis

- Rheumatoid arthritis

- Type II diabetes

- Hypersensitivity (environmental illness)

- Parkinson's

- Alzheimer's

- Chronic pain

- Bell's palsy

Prior to using hydrogen peroxide in my practice, I interviewed many patients, reviewed numerous clinical studies and read dozens of journal articles. Convinced of its benefits, I administered hydrogen peroxide orally using a thirty-five percent food grade H_2O_2 (one drop to eight ounces of water one to three times per day.) I gradually increased the dosage to fifteen to twenty drops per eight ounces of water with much success. Oral hydrogen peroxide is no longer recommended by the Bio-Oxidative Foundation due to the possibility of damage to the stomach wall.

While attending the International conference of Bio-Oxidative Medicine in Dallas, Texas, I discovered the many proven uses of *intravenous* hydrogen peroxide. In my opinion, intravenous hydrogen peroxide's greatest applications are the treatment of infections not responding to other medication and emphysema. Emphysema is very difficult to treat medically. With the medications that we presently have, the results are often less than desired. In the later stages of emphysema, the patients resort to using oxygen. I'm sure you have seen such patients walking with portable oxygen and nasal cannulas. This is a tragic sight that I would like to remedy if at all possible. In the majority of cases, I have found that intravenous hydrogen peroxide has met my highest expectations, including with a gentleman who had been on two to three liters of oxygen per minute for ten years. After only five treatments of intravenous hydrogen peroxide, he was able to put his oxygen tanks, tubes and regulator in storage.

Recently I treated a female patient diagnosed with Bell's palsy. I was amazed and elated when after only three treatments her Bell's palsy was cleared! Another patient noted a positive side effect; while taking the intravenous H_2O_2 for a different condition, he found that his enlarged prostate symptoms subsided.

Even though the American Medical Association does not approve of intravenous hydrogen peroxide and most insurance companies will not pay for such treatment, I implore you, as always, to research the literature, investigate the claims made for this treatment and decide for yourself whether or not intravenous hydrogen peroxide therapy should be added to your health care regimen.

Neurotherapy and Sclerotherapy (Prolotherapy)

One of my patients, a registered nurse, suffered from severe rheumatoid arthritis. Gus Prosch, M.D, subsequently treated her with neurotherapy and sclerotherapy. I became interested and visited him in his office. There he taught me the fundamentals of administering these injections. Neurotherapy consists of procaine and a small dose of long-acting cortisone injected precisely along a nerve. Neurotherapy can be used to alleviate a variety of pains; however, I've found it is most effective in treating osteoarthritis of the knee.

There are eight nerves surrounding the knee joint. When they become inflamed they cause the muscles to contract and. the joint movement becomes diminished. This puts pressure on the cartilage in the knee, thereby interfering with its circulation. The circulation in this joint is provided by osmosis. When you put pressure on the knee joint, it's like squeezing water from a sponge. By injecting in the nerves around the knee, you can immediately stop the pain. The injections may last several weeks and sometimes much longer. I have had a number of patients who were scheduled for knee surgery and after the injections their knees improved to the point at which they were able to forego the operation.

One of the first patients I treated with neurotherapy was my former mother-in-law. She had had one total knee replacement and was having similar symptoms in the other knee. She was scheduled for a second knee replacement. However, she stared experiencing heart trouble. At her age of eighty+, the surgeons didn't want to operate. She came for a visit and was only able to walk fifteen or twenty feet before stopping. I took her down to the office and gave her eight injections around the knee. They were somewhat painful, but she tolerated them well.

Within minutes, her pain was gone. After the injections, she went out shopping for three hours. Pretty good for a person who couldn't walk more than twenty feet! A year later I visited her and took more injections with me in case she needed them. She said she didn't! She is now 93 and her knee is still doing well. Another expensive, potentially dangerous, unnecessary surgery avoided by a nontraditional method.

Sclerotherapy or prolotherapy involves methods similar to neurotherapy but with a different focus. By injecting the tendon attachments to the bone with Pontocaine in a fifty-percent sugar solution, I can regenerate tendons and ligaments, which stabilizes the joint and greatly reduces pain and inflammation. This technique is very effective in treating persistent pain from stress joints such as ankles, knees, elbows and shoulders. Damaged ligaments and tendons that have not healed in six months can benefit from this treatment. Along with other patients successfully treated with this, sclerotherapy saved my son from knee surgery.

George Stuart Hackett, M. D., Of Canton, Ohio, spent years studying sclerotherapy. In 1956 he published *Ligament and Tendon Relaxation Treated by Prolotherapy*. He found that if the joint pain became aggravated with activity and improved with rest and heat, this type of therapy could be useful. The number of treatments depends on the ligaments involved, whether a large or small joint is involved, and the severity of the original injury.

The physicians of the American Osteopathic Academy of Sclerotherapy have carried on Dr. Hackett's work. Subsequently, a number of both D.O.s and M.D.s have been trained in this procedure in postgraduate seminars. Physical activity will improve muscle strength. However, since ligaments do not contain muscle fibers, more than exercise is needed for these injuries.

According to Dr. Proch, there are a number of indications for Sclerotherapy (Prolotherapy):

- Lax or torn ligaments associated with arthritis

- Joint pain lasting six weeks or longer

- Joint pain improved by a brace or support

- Joints that do not improve with manipulation

- Joints that are worse after surgery

- Joints that are better with rest and worse with exercise

- Joints that pop, snap or click

- Torn tendons or tendonitis that do not resolve after six weeks

Energy Medicine

I believe that energy medicine is the future of medicine. Contrary to what pharmaceutical companies would like us to believe, energy medicine will prove to be of far greater use than chemical medicine in the treatment of certain illnesses. Most illnesses are caused by a disruption in the frequencies of our electromagnetic field or our aura. Improper attitude, poor nutrition, exposure to pollution in the air, water and food can produce changes in our electromagnetic field. When we have a healthy electromagnetic field, we have a good immune system and are usually very healthy. However, alterations in the vibration pattern of our electromagnetic field can cause us problems.

Our bodies are electrical. Anything that lowers our frequency can cause illness. According to Dr. D.Gary Young, who has studied bio-electrical energy flow, our body frequency range is sixty-two to sixty-eight hertz. Our brain frequency increases by ten during the day and decreases by ten at night. Disease starts at fifty-eight hertz, influenza at fifty-seven, candida at fifty-five, Epstein Barr at fifty-two and cancer at forty-two. Energy healing methods today combine both new treatments and the re-introduction of age-old methods. Treatments for correcting imbalances in our electromagnetic field include the use of homeopathy, aromatherapy, thought field therapy, reike, therapeutic touch and radionics. I wholeheartedly recommend that you read *Vibrational Medicine*, by Richard Gerber, M.D., for a detailed study of most aspects of energy medicine.

There have been numerous delays in getting this book ready to publish. Now I think I know why. I have been told three times in the past year to read the book *Sanctuary,* and never found the time. Last week someone put a copy on my desk so I finally took the time to read it. When I did, I realized that I needed to discuss it briefly in my energy medicine section. The book discusses a therapy that Dr. Max Stevens researched and improved upon. He doesn't discuss disease per se, but he discusses energy, life force and spirit. He has further developed the therapy of "radionics." It is my belief that radionics was originated and developed by Galen Hieronymus. It was my privilege to meet and get to know this gentleman about 25 years ago before his death. He found that the frequency of an energy field could be determined from the hair or blood of an individual. He also discovered that he could also do it from a picture of the person. I was totally amazed and at first very skeptical. He discussed his research with me in detail and just before his death gave me three large cardboard boxes full of his research.

He proved that he could analyze a patient's energy frequencies from a picture and could "treat" the picture to readjust the patient's frequencies for better health. He also used this method to treat fields of agriculture to eliminate disease and increase crop yields.

With this background knowledge it was easy for me to understand "Dr. Max's" theory; radionics can be used both for good and evil, so one has to be extremely careful of the operator. I recommend that you also read *Sanctuary.* The next section on microcurrent therapy discusses another method of energy healing.

Microcurrent Therapy

Another fantastic use of energy is the microcurrent unit. We have used it with very good success but only for several months. Because my experience with it is limited, I have asked Julie Clemens to write this section to update you on this marvelous piece of equipment. I agree with Julie that you have to experience it to believe it.

Medicine has experimented with electrical application to the human body for 200 years. Every developed country has conducted research by various branches of medicine. The short version of all this research from all these countries has come to the same conclusion; less is better. Dr. Bjorn Nordenstrom, a renowned doctor and scientist in Sweden, has proved that human cellular activity is based on low-level electrical pulses and concludes that electrical stimulation can enhance the electrical activity of the basic building blocks of life, cellular activity.

To understand what microcurrent is, we need to define the word. It is an electrical measurement of "push," or power. We are all familiar with the measurement of "amps," correctly known as amperage. The average power in a regular household circuit is ten "amp" service. So an amp is a lot of power if ten of them combined can power the electrical needs of one zone in the average American home.

When we take one amp and divide it into 1,000 units of power, that is called a mili-amp. Mathematically it looks like this: $1/1,000^{th}$. When we divide the amp into 1,000,000 units of power, we now have a micro-amp, or $1/1,000,000^{th}$ of an amp, which is a very tiny amount of power.

Research proves that microcurrent applications enter the cells. This brings about cellular stimulation at the deepest level of healing. There is little if any sensation connected to microcurrent, as the "power" is so small as it enters the cell. This level of electrical push is lower than most people's ability to feel it.

Electrical stimulation in medicine today is best known in the use of the Transcutaneous Electrical Neuro Stimulation (T.E.N.S.). This device is used for interrupting the signals from the brain to the body that communicate to the body that pain is present. A T.E.N.S. unit is used when traditional medical solutions for pain elimination have been used without success. The T.E.N.S. unit is strapped to the outside of the body or, in cases of severe chronic pain, the unit is surgically installed under the skin. This device has no corrective properties.

In a study conducted by the University of Washington, cotton sponges were inserted under the skins of laboratory rats. After twenty-one days, collagen had totally surrounded the sponge, thus creating a barrier around the sponge. When microcurrent was used to deliver frequencies to this area, the collagen dissipated and allowed energy to flow normally once more.

The conclusion by the researchers conducting these tests is that these frequencies applied by microcurrent break down the fibrosis processes in the body. This eliminates scars, as well as all types and manner of fibrosis in the body, and allows the electrical circuitry of the body to operate properly again. Traditional medicine certainly doesn't deny that there are myriad electrical forces at work within the body, in addition to chemical ones exerted by hormones and enzymes and physical ones like the pressure of the blood in the arteries and veins. Every human thought and action is accompanied by the conduction of electrical signals along the fibers of the nervous system. Indeed, life wouldn't exist at all without a constant flow of ions across the membranes of cells.

The idea that electric currents can stimulate bodily repair, alert defense mechanisms, and control the growth and function of cells is not new in medicine. Bioelectromagnetics dates back at least 200 years. But this entire field of research and exploration got a doubtful reputation at the turn of the century, when researchers of that day proposed electromagnetism as a panacea and were proved wrong. A stigma has been attached to electrical devices in medicine ever since.

One of the most astounding findings of modern research has been the ability of microcurrent to reverse fibrosis. There are many types and forms of fibrosis in various named disease conditions. Emphysema is one of the most dramatic. The lungs lose elasticity and become like leather, until they no longer allow the contraction and expansion of lung tissue. Eventually, the diaphragm stops working and the body ceases function without air.

One story of emphysema recovery happened in Seattle. A man with emphysema was told by his doctor that his days were numbered. It was only a matter of time until his lungs would stop functioning. This man purchased a microcurrent frequency computer. He used the frequency program that was used in the Rat Skin study that reverses the fibrosis process. Some months later the man was on the golf course and ran into his doctor. The doctor was startled to see him and said, "What are you doing here? I thought you were dead!"

A first hand experience of mine involves a woman from Colorado in the last stages of emphysema. I had done telephone nutritional counseling with her some months prior to her call to me in January 1999. She called and informed me that her doctor said she only had a couple of months to live. She was on many pharmaceutical drugs as well as oxygen, and she fought for each breath she took. I took the attitude that she had nothing to lose by trying something new. I had only read research at this time about "normalizing" fibrosis conditions, but with impending death, just what did she have to lose?

She purchased a microcurrent computer designed for home use. Her next contact came about seven months later. She was elated about her improving ability to breathe. She told me she had immersed herself in the bathtub while applying the frequencies to her entire body. She related that she had never returned to her doctor, had stopped all medications and that after about four months of spending hours in the bathtub daily, she was able to breathe on her own without the assistance of oxygen. She was walking to her mailbox. That is nothing short of a miraculous response.

With microcurrent, some of the conditions we accept as "incurables" now become treatable and in many cases reversed.

The microcurrent story at its finest level must include Jim Suzuki. My meeting him is where my personal experience with this technology began in 1998. He was born in Seattle, Washington. In 1959 he entered the U. S. Air Force navigator school. His military job became launching missiles from Florida. He graduated from the University of Washington in 1958 with an Electronic Engineer degree.

Jim returned to Seattle and began his career as an engineer for the Boeing Aircraft Company in their Aerospace division. His job was testing the function of missile systems. He designed and developed a test system to determine the susceptibility of the Minuteman Missile System to the EMP nuclear explosion.

He was also designing a test system for the Boeing Advanced SST, when the contract was cancelled three years into the program.

Jim worked on the ALCM cruise missile program. He designed and developed a test for this system. He became chief troubleshooter for all cruise missiles in the United States. In all of these test design assignments, the frequency response of the system was the most important and useful. In subsequent years, Jim would use that knowledge and relate it to the human body.

His interest in microcurrent started when he got a "bad" back. He followed the traditional medical routine of pain pills and muscle relaxants. He consulted a specialist and was scheduled for back surgery. During the course of pre-surgical paperwork, Jim met the head orthopedic surgeon of the hospital. This man walked with the same slow, stooped posture that Jim was forced to adopt due to pain. When he asked this doctor what was the matter with his back, the doctor responded "the same thing as yours." The doctor explained the downside of back surgery and informed Jim that he himself had chosen not to participate in what he explained was all too often the first of a series of surgeries. He said that most back surgeries did not work, and often did not relieve pain. This alarmed Jim, and he cancelled his plans for surgery.

Jim continued with pain and moved with difficulty. In the meantime, he discovered kinesiology. This is Jim's area of expertise. He incorporated this knowledge into his microcurrent muscle frequencies. He designed programs that duplicate the normal function of healthy muscles. When he applied these frequencies using microcurrent as the power to deliver these frequencies to his own back, the pain stopped. He has had no back problems since. All his training was now combined to design an easy method for everyone to use microcurrent.

He has to date duplicated the normal frequencies emitted by the organs, muscles, normal fluid flow, bone regeneration, gum disease, tissue regeneration, tissue anesthesia, swelling and programs that duplicate emotional stability. When these normal frequencies are applied to abnormal conditions, the body responds by returning to normal functioning. He has designed over 400 applications for the human body. He places these frequencies in programs to duplicate the way the body works. A miniature computer powered by batteries runs the programs. Microcurrent is the delivery method.

He had so much success with correcting unsolvable problems that he just kept conducting more experiments. He started making these computers for others to use. His results excited everyone who encountered this new technology. He needed money to continue his experiments and began selling these computers to people overseas.

One of the frequencies proved to be mysterious in its action. When applied to the origin and insertion of a muscle, the muscle became "normal" in length and elasticity. To rephrase that, every muscle begins at a bone (origin), and tucks under other muscles (insertion). As muscles are engaged for movement, the muscle contracts and the opposing muscle relaxes, thus allowing the engaged muscle to expand. Energy moving through the muscle allows this to happen. When we transpose the word *frequency* for *energy* we expand our understanding of this event.

During his experiments, he had created a frequency band that would make a muscle normal in all aspects. A band is a range of many frequencies within a given set of parameters or highs and lows. This frequency corrects loose, flaccid muscles to resume their proper tension. When a muscle is too tight (and therefore painful) the muscles resume normal flexion and tension, which results in less pain. This single discovery led him to develop a series of frequencies, arranged in a program that firms muscles of the face. When applied in sequence, this gives the muscles tone and elasticity that become lost with the aging process. He had developed the equivalent to a non-surgical face-lift. The muscle-firming procedure that worked for the face translated well into the larger muscles of the body. Programs were designed to firm the breasts, arms, abdomen, thighs, and buttocks. The proper frequencies for these muscle groups result in a tightening action that firms flaccid muscles. The treatment takes minutes, and there are no side effects. It makes muscles firm again. Everyone wants to look good and feel good.

This was an avenue to earn money that was needed to continue his experiments. The dreary process of application for patents requires a lot of money. He retired from the Boeing Company and now devotes his full attention to microcurrent research, development, and manufacture. He manufactures these computers and trains Cosmetologists and Aestheticians in how to use them. His company sells his beauty computers in the U.S. and in sixteen foreign countries. Microcurrent Frequency Computers sells the medical and home use computers in the United States.

Research using microcurrent for all types of conditions has been conducted all over the world. Countless articles have been published in medical and health trade magazines. There is a lot of information available from the development stages through the 1980s from physical therapists in Seattle and Portland, Oregon. Many health professionals have used various models of microcurrent computers as they were developed. The scientific research is found in publications such as *The Journal of*

American Medicine, (JAMA) and *Lancet,* the medical journal from the United Kingdom. Libraries and the Internet are good sources for research articles.

Dr. Bjorn Nordenstrom is the most renowned doctor in Sweden. He pioneered a series of remarkable innovations in clinical radiology that seemed radical at the time but are now routinely employed at every major hospital in the world. He was promoted to the most respected position in his field, head of diagnostic radiology in Stockholm's Karolinska Institute, then the pre-eminent radiological research laboratory in the world. In 1985 he served as chairman of Karolinska's Nobel Assembly, which chooses the Nobel laureates in medicine. In 1983, he published a book of his experimental work covering 20 years of research. It is called *Biologically Closed Electric Circuits: Clinical, Experimental and Theoretical Evidence for an Additional Circulatory System.*

Dr. Nordenstrom's discoveries explain how an injury, an infection, a tumor, or even normal activity of the organs switches on the body's electrical system. His work explains how the electric currents course through arteries and veins and across capillary walls, drawing white blood cells and metabolic compounds into and out of surrounding tissues. This electrical system works to balance the activity of internal organs, and in the case of injuries represents the very foundation of the healing process. Researchers in France, Italy and Japan are beginning to duplicate his experiments.

American medical colleagues of Nordenstrom say his work is undeniable revolutionary. The mystery is that the rank and file of the American medical community has not noticed that Nordenstrom's theories exist. If you ask cancer experts, biophysicists, or pathologists—scientists whose disciplines are the heart and soul of Nordenstrom's book—you probably will get a blank stare with the response, "Bjorn who?" Medical researchers, like everyone else, tend to move with the current fads in medicine. If something is not backed by an enormous amount of money and loud press, they tend to ignore it. Researchers who generally learn something as a "truth" don't like to hear that they based a large part of their careers on things that were either incomplete or not completely correct. So microcurrent has gone overseas for it's research proofs and trials. The Internet has a glut of research data. There is an address at the end of this section for anyone who desires further research information on microcurrent. This worldwide database increases rapidly.

Over the years of learning to use microcurrent and its application to the body, medical professionals in all areas of health care have contributed. Chiropractors, massage therapists, orthopedic surgeons, physical therapists and naturopaths have all played a part in developing protocols and procedures. Each set of professional applications added new insights into microcurrent use. There is a huge difference in equipment from company to company that manufacture microcurrent units. Most use simple microcurrent electrical charge. These units get results. To use microcurrent that delivers normal frequencies emitted by the body is the difference between a scooter and a car. When the programs are delivered with kinesiology incorporated into the delivery to duplicate the way the body works, you have results that are unbelievable.

It was during the process of developing these procedures that the mystery of the muscles "connectedness" began to unfold. While working to correct the Temporal-Mandibular Joint muscles (TMJ), a whole new level of understanding evolved. When the muscle attachments surrounding the ear, neck and skull bones are "normalized" in conjunction with five specific muscle attachments within the mouth, a whole series of adjustments happen throughout the entire body. It appears that the muscles of the upper body pull on and support the muscles in the shoulders and back, which in turn pull and support all the muscles down to and including the sacrum. The sacrum is the "keystone" of the spine. It adjusts to all types of muscle changes throughout the entire muscular and skeletal structure. When muscle tension in the jaw area is adjusted to normal conditions, there is a domino effect throughout all the muscles. The uppermost muscles of the body, having come to normal function and tension, release undue strain on the supporting muscles of the shoulders and back. After an adjustment of these muscles, the entire body adjusts over the following days.

Many muscle problems disappear entirely in as little as three sessions of adjustment with the microcurrent unit. This procedure is called the *upper body release*. Most people are sufficiently realigned in structure to have the second session performed within one week. During this second session of muscle correction, the jaw muscles are checked to insure that they are holding the adjustment in proper tension. Now the foundation of the body is addressed. The feet are adjusted to resume their original structure. All the muscles are treated from the knees down to the soles of the foot. These corrections also translate up to the sacrum. The body responds to these lower muscle adjustments by adapting on its own with the muscles of the feet in normal alignment with the rest of the body. After this is done, the body makes further changes due to the proper muscle balance of the feet.

The third session in this series of treatments is a recheck of all the muscle adjustments done by the previous two sessions and now identifies the changes that were automatically made by the body as a result of the treatments. At this time, if there are muscles that have not corrected themselves, the therapist places each muscle into correct position and adjusts tension by application of the proper frequency program. At this time all the muscles in the body have been adjusted to normal placement and pain is gone in most cases.

This has far-reaching benefits for everyone who experiences pain. Back pain is the number one reason for lost work by the American worker. When pain is relieved, all the muscle-relaxing drugs can be replaced by the microcurrent application to muscles. When pain is from sprain, strain or injury, then the muscle repair program can be applied. When a muscle is strained and out of tension, especially at joint connections, pain is experienced. Microcurrent is able to shorten the sagging and loose muscles and lengthen the painful tight muscle, thus relieving pain in most cases. Very seldom are surgery or other heroic measures necessary to relieve joint pain. When the muscles are adjusted to proper placement and function, the pain ceases. Athletes around the globe have been eager to embrace the use of microcurrent, with notable results.

The subject of athletes brings our microcurrent story to China in 1988. Jim Suzuki has a partner in each country where he sells his computers. In China this person is Dr. Tat Chee Tam. He went to a hotel near the Asian Games Village, giving free demonstration treatments. He relieved *tendonitis* that had been bothering Beijing Mayor Chen Xitong, and worked on Vice Mayor Zhang Haifa. They were greatly impressed.

Soon after his work with these politicians, he was summoned to work on a long-standing ailment for Wan Li, head of the National People's Congress Standing Committee, an office of power and influence second only to the leader of all China. Dr. Tam quickly and painlessly relieved Mr. Wan Li of his long-standing bout with pain. Dr. Tam explained the many uses of microcurrent. Mr. Wan Li summoned Mr. Chen and Mr. Zhang, the key organizers of the Olympic Games being held in Beijing. They were impressed so thoroughly that Dr. Tam and Jim Suzuki were appointed medical consultants to the Chinese Asian Games Team.

The results of those games are history now. The Chinese won half the gold medals in the thirty-seven-nation competition. The Olympic committee checked all Chinese athletes for steroid use, while Jim and Dr. Tam were in the athlete's locker rooms balancing their muscles prior to performance.

Needless to say, Mr. Wan Li was very grateful to Jim Suzuki. He asked what China could do for him, to repay his services to the Chinese athletes. Jim did not hesitate in his request. It takes many hundreds of thousands of dollars to conduct clinical trials on any medical device in the United States, which is necessary for federal drug agency approval. The details and costs of trials on humans in a medical setting and in the numbers required to establish effectiveness in America is staggering for a small business.

Clinical trials were to be conducted at the University of Beijing following the guidelines from the United States Food and Drug Asministration (FDA). This is how the microcurrent frequency computers accomplished the clinical trails required by the FDA. The microcurrent frequency computers are FDA approved for Lymph edema and Fibromyalgia. This resulted in the Hospitals and Clinics in China becoming some of the best customers of professional Microcurrent Frequency Computers.

The grapevine of health care professionals also tells the story of Carl Lewis and Ben Johnson at the Seoul Olympics. Three days before the race to see who was the fastest runner, Ben Johnson was suffering from a tight hamstring muscle. The injury was severe enough to keep Johnson from competing in the race. Carl Lewis loaned Johnson his microcurrent computer and showed him how to use it to repair and lengthen the tight muscles. The rest is history. Ben Johnson beat Carl Lewis in competition as the fastest runner. Joe Montana, star quarterback of the San Francisco 49ers, is said to have used microcurrent therapy to assist his amazing recovery in returning to play just two weeks after back surgery. The Chinese gymnast Chen Cuiting, who won two gold medals at the Seoul Olympics and three more at the Asian Games, says that two of those medals would have been impossible for her to win without microcurrent frequency therapy.

ATP Reactions to Microcurrent

The necleotide adenosine triphosphate (ATP) is an organic molecule that stores and releases chemical energy for use in body cells. It is the main source of energy in cells as it stores chemical energy in a form that cells can use. ATP temporarily stores the energy-consuming reactions in the cell, as its bonds are broken. This is released to provide the raw energy of bodily action. For example, when a runner has used all the ATP available, he has to stop. He has used up the "energy" available to allow action by the muscles.

By normalizing cell activity, inflammation is reduced while collagen-producing cells are increased. Healthy cell metabolism results in a healthy, pain-free internal environment. The small numbers of micro amps used in microcurrent therapy is sensation-free. Medical practitioners have long understood electrical exchanges within the body. Applying that knowledge has been slow in developing. Doctors and physical therapists all over the world have been using microcurrent to heal injured muscles, tendons, wounds and myriad of injuries and ailments for the past twenty years. It has not been available to the general public, due to the lack of FDA approval (that now exists).

In 1982 Dr. N. Cheng did a study to determine whether higher currents or lower currents produced the most beneficial effects. He measured ATP levels in rat skin cells that had been stimulated with only sixty to 500 microamperes of electricity, then ATP levels that had been stimulated with currents from 1,000 to 5,000 micro amperes. He found that ATP levels increased by as much as 500% when stimulated with only sixty amperes. The cell showed no ATP increase at all when stimulated with 1,000 microamperes. The "magic" level was determined to increase ATP. It was during this same study that it was proved that the frequencies delivered by the microcurrent break down fibrosis conditions. This eliminates scars regardless of how old, and all other fibrotic conditions. That makes microcurrent viable to treat many "untreatable" conditions that have fibrosis, such as emphysema, fibroid cysts and tumors, M.S., ALS, and more.

The external addition of microcurrent will increase the production of ATP, protein synthesis, oxygenation, ion exchange, absorption of nutrients and elimination of waste products, and neutralizes the oscillating polarity of deficient cells. Thus homeostasis is restored.

Stimulation of ATP within mitochondria resumes vigorous cellular function. Infection and other foreign bodies can be resisted and repelled. The delivery of frequency is very simple. When a body is placed in water, the frequencies travel through the water and the wet body absorbs the frequencies. Most unsupervised programs are applied with water application, such as having the patient in a tub of water with the electrodes in the water.

A recent publication by Dr. Edward C. Kondrot, M.D., titled *Miracle Eye Cures with Microcurrent* details the results of using microcurrent application for reversal of eye conditions. The units he describes have dials for tuning specific single frequencies for eye treatments. The complicated delivery method of these single frequencies leads to the conclusion that one needs a professional to apply these treatments or a great deal of information on application of frequencies to the body. It also verifies the complete frequency programs of the normal function of the eyes through the microcurrent frequency programs I have been using. The amazing results outlined in this chapter equal our results. Our delivery method is as simple as pushing two buttons. The treatment takes no professional assistance. The therapy is delivered in pre-programmed sessions at home. The microcurrent frequency computers use a pair of glasses with pinhole lenses for the frequency programs to be administered through special contact points where the glasses touch around the eye lenses and behind the ears. It is easy to wear glasses that allow you to see well enough to continue normal activity while the eye program runs. This program reverses macular degeneration, myopia, cataracts and glaucoma.

Let's look at the medical indications for microcurrent use. These uses have been tested and proven with research and clinical application thus far. I'll separate the uses into groups, so you understand the similarities in response. First is the *straight minute electrical stimulation of microcurrent alone.* Straight microcurrent is where worldwide research has been conducted. Next are the *normal frequencies of the body* that have been duplicated and are delivered by using microcurrent as the power. To my knowledge, the microcurrent frequency computer is the only one on the market at this point in time that uses these normal frequencies.

There are powerful innovative procedures that utilize the abilities of the combination of normal frequencies and microcurrent applied in effective treatments that bring astounding results. These require the assistance of health professionals. Dr. Gene Schroeder at his Rainbow Wellness Clinic in Prescott, Arizona, is one of the cutting-edge doctors that offer these treatments. The school that trains health professionals in the application and use of microcurrent is the Northwest Institute of Natural Therapies in Sandpoint, Idaho. Treatments to correct conditions such as TMJ, Scoliosis, Chronic Fatigue, MS, Parkinson's and other complex conditions require special training, with considerable knowledge of the anatomy and physiology of the body.

The following section contains medical conditions that have been effectively treated with microcurrent. These are almost with-out exception treatable without side effects or sensation. There is, of course, always the exception to the rule. I have performed treatments for severe conditions that in the ordinary person would be totally sensation-free. In the case of long-standing and severe conditions there is always a myriad of variable symptoms to consider. For instance most people with *arthritis* simply apply the specific frequencies that break down the calcium deposits and treat the pain with no sensation. At the other end of the spectrum are the two people I encountered that had such severe deposits that they experienced discomfort as the deposits broke up and they required the assistance of the pain for hands program to be taken directly after the arthritis program. *Abdominal cramps* and other types of pain also respond differently with various individuals. One neighbor of mine experienced *migraines* every day of her life. She eliminated the headaches after two months of home care. The choice is home treatment versus professional care. The price of the home unit quickly equals that of professional care.

Scoliosis and TMJ problems require professionally administered therapy sessions to correct. Professionally applied treatments are always needed with the italicized conditions below.

Acute pain, *Bell's Palsy,* bone degeneration, bone growth, body lifts, burns, *bursitis, capsulitis, chronic fatigue, chronic pain, Carpal tunnel, disc disease, decubitus ulcers, edema and lymph edema,* eye focus, cataracts, macular degeneration, emphysema, gum disease, hair growth, face lift, *Fibromyalgia, Fibromyalgia occurrence reduction,* fibrosis, fibrosis occurrence reduction, Injuries, Intertracable pain, *Lymph flow increase, myofacial pain, Myositis,* Migraines, muscle repair, *Neuropathies, Pre and Post operation conditioning, reduce swelling, Rotor cuff problems, Scoliosis, Sciatica, Sinus conditions, Stroke rehabilitation,* soft tissue repair, surgical incisions, *Synovitis, Tendonitis, T.M.J. syndrome, Whiplash and wound healing.* WHEW!

That list is simply too good to be true, right? Well that was my first impression and I became quite skeptical as the list grew, as do most health practitioners. Hair growth and fibromyalgia? But when you compare what all these conditions have in common, and couple that with what microcurrent does best, then it makes perfect sense.

In 1999 I was treating a patient for psoriasis with homeopathy. She had battled this for twenty-eight years. She was depressed, mentally foggy and physically exhausted most of the time. She came to me with a recent outbreak of lesions on her hands and legs. I gave the appropriate remedy at the correct potency.

Sometimes with homeopathy care, the body expels the condition. This is called an "aggravation." This is when the body responds to the remedy with a sudden and exuberant reaction. It's as if there exists a dam of suppression holding the condition inside the body. The remedy is given, and this invisible dam breaks and there is a blessed expulsion from built-up pressure from years of suppressive therapies. When this happened to this lady, her body chose the newest lesion on her leg to expel volumes of yellow-green infection and mucus. This lesion grew to the size of a softball on her calf. It was very painful for her.

She lived in a remote area alone in the forest. Despite her pain, I talked her into coming down her mountain. I was surprised to find the degree of severity of the lesion. I cleaned what had become a sizeable ulcer, and we applied several different frequency programs to make her comfortable. A leg pain frequency was applied first. This temporarily made her more comfortable. She could hardly walk due to the severity of discomfort. The pain was much better after a few minutes, application of the pain program. I switched to the leg ulcer program.

We both watched in amazement. We could actually see tissue at the deepest part of the ulcer become a healthy pink color.

I kept her under observation for the next three days. During this time we watched as the microcurrent frequencies stimulated new tissue regeneration. We could actually discern this as it happened. It was like watching a speeded up time-frame photo series, like those one sees on the nature programs as flowers open and the sun sets at a rapid pace. We were and still are in awe of what we witnessed together watching this large ulcer form new tissue before our eyes.

Another amazement to me was the response by an elderly A.L.S. patient. I applied frequency therapy on her muscles for an hour and a half. When I was finished with the treatment, she was able to form recognizable words. Her muscles were relaxed, in normal tension on her upper body. She was more flexible and sat comfortably. She was also able to expand her lungs for easier breathing. The next morning, she reported that she was able to sleep through the night without the aid of oxygen for the first time in five years.

I can relate three years worth of these little miracles. I can relate one story after another. So can every person that has used microcurrent frequency computers. The health providers who have worked with this can all tell the same types of stories. They love their computers, for nothing in their experience works on the "untreatable" conditions with such wonderful results and lack of side effects. The people that own home computers get used to using them on a daily basis. They are healthier. Every day they use their computers for *burns* from cooking, the *bruises* the kids get, *circulation improvement, high blood pressure and depression.* The only thing I can say to people who think I'm hooked on frequency use is this: You gotta see it to believe it. The results of this therapy get referrals from everyone who experiences it.

References
Web site of research contact numbers for more information on microcurrent. The Northwest Institute of Natural Therapies, 986 Beers Humbird Rd., Sagle, Idaho, 83860. Phone: 208-265-2666.

Foot Reflexology

There are points in your body, primarily the hands, feet and ears, that correspond to various organs in your body. You can make a diagnosis by pressing these specific points. If the points are tender, there's a likelihood that the organ system they relate to has a problem. I used foot reflexology extensively in the mid-seventies before I switched to kinesiology. Kinesiology is more accurate, but foot reflexology can still be important in medical evaluation.

A female patient came to the emergency room complaining of upper abdominal distress. In the process of examining her I decided that she would benefit from foot reflexology. I identified a problem with her right ovary and told her that she should followup with her own physician. She called a month later, telling me how happy she had become by consenting to foot reflexology. Her physician discovered an ovarian cancer that may not have been found without the technique.

Yet another female patient was hospitalized with a fever of undetermined origin. Regardless of the number of tests, we were unable to locate the source of her infection. We did urine tests, blood tests, X-rays, and so forth, all to no avail. One day, while making rounds, I demonstrated foot reflexology on this patient to an internal medicine specialist. The results indicated that she had a kidney infection even though all her urine tests were negative. We subsequently ordered another urine culture and ultimately isolated the problem. Without foot reflexology, it probably would have taken us longer to arrive at the diagnosis.

On a lighter note, I was at a local watering hole talking to a young lady. After a while, the conversation turned to health matters and I jokingly told her I was a veterinarian. I claimed that veterinarians were better diagnosticians than physicians because we could check a person's foot to make a diagnosis. She became very skeptical and scoffed, "If you can tell what's wrong with me, I'll buy you a beer!" She claimed it was a chronic problem and didn't think I could tell her what it was. I checked her foot and quickly told her she had a chronic urinary problem. She was so surprised that she just about fell off the barstool, but I did get my beer.

One evening at a staff meeting at our clinic in Ishpeming, Dr. Williams developed a severe headache. He decided to cancel the meeting because of the headache; however, I persuaded him to let me do foot kinesiology on him. Within 15 minutes his headache was gone and we were able to conduct the meeting.

Recently my wife had several episodes of severe spasmodic coughing that was not helped by using cough preparations. The only thing that stopped her coughing in the middle of the night was rubbing the lung parts on the bottom of her feet!

I had a number of patients in Michigan who firmly believed in foot reflexology. They not only tested, but also treated themselves on a prophylactic basis by massaging their feet. Foot reflexology is another modality to add to your ever-expanding health care world. There are a number of books on the subject.

Urine Therapy

Occasionally, I suggest that a patient use a very effective therapy that doesn't cost a penny! I try to intuitively screen my patients before I recommend this therapy. I'm sure that most would not consider trying it because of preconceived erroneous ideas. *Your Own Perfect Medicine* by Martha Christy or *The Water Of Life* by J. W. Armstrong are two excellent books explaining this therapy. I am referring to urine therapy, a treatment backed by over seventy years of medical research.

Thousands of patients have been healed, sometimes of an incurable disease, with urine therapy. I have had good success with this treatment method, but I don't prescribe it to my patients often enough. A few conditions that benefit from urine therapy are allergy, infection, colitis, Crohn's disease, chronic fatigue syndrome, constipation, weight loss, malaria, gangrene, fungus and dermatitis.

Urine is not dirty. It is sterile and full of very helpful products such as hormones, insulin, antibodies, enzymes, brain chemicals, DHEA, melatonin, vitamins and minerals plus dozens of other compounds. It should not be considered disgusting but appreciated for its therapeutic value. I have used urea, the main component of urine, extensively for treating glaucoma and lymphedema. Some doctors administer it by injection. Others combine it with homeopathic medicinals.

I find that the easiest method is to drink several ounces of urine daily to maintain perfect health. Much larger amounts are used to treat an illness. In severe cases, good results have been obtained by having the patient drink *all* of their urine until they improve. Specific dietary advice has to be given to each patient. In some cases, fasting is also necessary. If prescription medication is taken at the same time, expect limited improvement.

Today I had a ten-year-old boy come in as a new patient. Two days ago his mother called and asked if I could help him. He had a viral infection of his eyes and had been to see three ophthalmologists and she had spent over $800 on medication without any benefit. I told her to put several drops of urine in each eye every three to four hours. Today, on examination I could find only minimal conjunctivitis and his mother claimed that his eyes were improved over sixty percent! I then did kinesiology on him. The urine therapy was working. Kinsiology indicated that olive leaf extract would be of further aid in eliminating the virus. He also tested to be low in L-phenylalame and B vitamins that would help his attention deficit disorder so he could do better in school. Another big plus for kinesiology testing and urine therapy!

Hugs

I believe in them and give them to most of my patients. Unfortunately, not everyone appreciates them as much as I do. I keep two "Hugs Posters" in each of my examining rooms. I think you might enjoy them. I do not know the authors but I extend to them my gratitude for their thoughts. Hugs are great medicine.

"HUGS"

It's wondrous what a hug can do,

A hug can cheer your when you're blue.

A hug can say, "I love you so"

Or, "Gee, I hate to see you go."

A hug is "welcome back again,"

And great to see you! Where've you been?

A hug can soothe a small child's pain

And bring a rainbow after rain.

The hug! There's just no doubt about it.

We scarcely could survive without it!

A hug delights and warms and charms,

It must be why God gave us arms.

Hugs are great for fathers and mothers,

Sweet for sisters, swell for brothers,

And chances are your favorite aunts

Love them more than potted plants.

Kittens crave them. Puppies love them.

Heads of state are not above them.

A hug can break the language barrier

And make your travels so much merrier.

No need to fret about your store of 'em,

The more you give the more there's more of 'em.

So stretch those arms without delay

And GIVE SOMEONE A HUG TODAY!

"HERE'S TO HUGS"

Hugs keep you healthy,

Hugs can relieve pain and depression,

Reduce stress, help overcome fear,

Are invigorating, rejuvenating

And just plain feel good.

Hugs are all natural

They require no special equipment

Do not harm the environment

Are naturally sweet with no sugar or artificial sweeteners.

Hugs are perfect

There are no parts to wear out, no monthly payments

You can never have too many and they always fit

Hugs are theft-proof

Low-energy consumption and high-energy yield

And fully recyclable.

Hugs make happy days happier and impossible days possible!

Chapter 6

Health Issues for the
New Millennium

The future of creation is threatened by activity that does little to improve the human condition. Nowhere is this more apparent than in health problems hampered by a profit-driven economy. Two examples are cancer and mercury/root canals.

In spite of a world order that is based on control and monopoly, alternative and effective therapies have emerged. These therapies are the seeds of change that will carry us on the right path as we enter a new millennium.

Cancer

Cancer has been a major health problem for many years despite spending vast amounts of research time and money. The American Cancer Society spends eighty-four percent of donations on overhead. Only sixteen percent of donations go to cancer-related problems. It is true we have experienced some limited success using the "Big Three" of surgery, radiation and chemotherapy. However, these treatments fail all too often. We need to research ways to improve the immune system rather than wasting resources trying to find a new drug. Louis Pasteur has been given credit for our current germ therapy; however; on his deathbed he confessed, "The pathogen (the invading threat) is nothing. The terrain (environment/immune system) is everything!"

Physicians are often forced into using the "Big Three" methods of treatments (cut, burn and poison) advocated by the state medical society. In California, it's illegal to treat cancer patients with anything but the "Big Three." I have already told you about the Black Herbal Ointment I have been forbidden to use even though it is almost one-hundred percent effective for skin cancer. In many states, doctors have been treated like criminals for using natural remedies that work and save you money.

In the 1930s Royal Raymond Rife developed a method to cure deadly diseases—even cancer. He used "energy medicine." Rife found that he could eliminate disease by determining the body's electromagnetic frequency and altering it by using the opposite resonance frequency. His work was so amazing that Rife was awarded fourteen government contracts to develop practical uses. One of his most remarkable accomplishments was a very powerful microscope enabling him to study bacteria and viruses in the living state. He found that microorganisms differed depending on their environment.

Rife also suggested that microorganisms could change form and character by changing their environment. Approximately ninety percent of the bacterial flora cells in our body are located in the intestines. Now, how do you feel knowing this? Fortunately, these intestinal flora bacteria are necessary for good health. They detoxify cancer-causing chemicals in our system and produce vitamins and other essential factors that we need to stay healthy. I believe that if the intestinal environment becomes unhealthy, the bacteria can mutate from a beneficial bacteria to a pathological form. Many prominent medical doctors of the period confirmed his method and cures. Unfortunately, I believe that the government and the medical profession felt they would lose a lot of money if such methods were used. His inventions were destroyed and Royal Rife was ruined.

Please take some time and read *The Cancer Cure That Worked*, by Barry Lynes. I'm sure the achievements of Royal Rife will capture your imagination. I'm also sure you'll be offended by the injustice he suffered. Many have tried to duplicate Rife's equipment. There are a number of different versions you can buy at a variety of prices. I understand that some of them work very well; some do not.

The FDA has not approved the different versions of Rife's equipment. A medical researcher acquaintance of mine recently developed a prototype of Rife's equipment and so far his results in treating cancer have been very encouraging. If you decide you want to purchase one to heal a loved one, please investigate them in depth before you select a unit.

Again, I want to emphasize that in the process of affecting a cure for cancer, I believe without question that the parasite infection I find with every cancer patient must be treated promptly to take the load off the immune system. Clearing the parasites will result in a much higher "cure rate" for any cancer. If the cancer is of any size, I believe that it should also be surgically removed (if possible) to again take a load off the immune system. If additional medical evaluation indicates that radiation or chemotherapy is advisable, I would prefer radiation if possible. I believe that chemotherapy suppresses the immune system and that should be avoided if at all possible.

In addition to eliminating the parasites, I believe that there are other alternative means of fighting cancer that can be used in conjunction with traditional allopathic methods. I would suggest that you get second opinions from alternative practitioners. Some complementary treatments for cancer that I have found to be beneficial are:

- Vitamin C
- MGN 3
- Coffee enemas
- Visualization
- Vitamin A and B12
- Essiac Tea
- Black Salve
- Pancreatic enzymes
- Flax seed oil/cottage cheese mixture
- Zinc oratate
- Aromatherapy

These are just a few of the alternative cancer treatments. There are many more.

For any serious illness I advise getting two or three medical opinions. Remember, two heads are better than one—even if one is a pumpkin head!

Mercury/Root Canals

Throughout this book, I have emphasized the need to keep our immune system healthy. One way to do so is to avoid the things that adversely affect our immune system. This brings up a very controversial subject here in the United States, dental fillings of silver and mercury and root canals. I am definitely concerned about the possible side effects in some but not all individuals. However, my dentist firmly believes that they are safe. Unfortunately, I have not been able to change her mind or get her to read any of the considerable available information on these subjects.

Many people are sensitive to even low doses of mercury exposure. It attacks various organ systems of the body. I have many patients with multiple complaints that have been helped by removing the mercury from their bodies. One of the first things to consider in a patient who has symptoms due to mercury toxicity is removing the causative agents. In many cases this means removing dental fillings. However, in the process of removing the fillings, some patients get worse. One way to help avoid this is to give the patient several EDTA Chelation treatments during the removal of the fillings.

We are all exposed to more toxins and pollution as each year goes by. Among the most dangerous of these is mercury. It is considered to be toxic at any concentration in the body. It can cause a very wide range of disturbances such as nerve and muscle problems, mood changes, problems with organ systems and general problems such as fatigue and weakness. It has been confused with MS.

Oral ingestion is often not a problem unless large doses are involved. The real problem in the mercury is with the vapor phase, as it can cross the blood brain barrier and cause damage to brain cells thus resulting in memory loss, poor concentration, irritability, fits of anger and dental problems.

I advise my patients not to get mercury fillings and/or to remove them if present, as mercury is so toxic to all human organisms that there can be cell death or irreversible chemical damage long before clinically observable symptoms appear. After placement of mercury and silver fillings, there is a persistent low-level release of metallic mercury vapor into the body for many years.

Mercury toxicity appears to have a direct causal relationship to the development of allergic sensitivity to foods, chemicals and other environmental factors. And yet the American Dental Association denies that mercury fillings are associated with human illness despite all the scientific data to the contrary.

Tyler Co. has an oral formula to detox mercury that is very helpful and contains n-acetyl-cysteine, L-cysteine, reduced L-gluthathione, vitamin E and selenium. Jonathan Wright, M.D. has discovered that when many companies took the lead out of paints because of its toxic effects, they replaced the lead with mercury! Now isn't that just dandy? It's like replacing a 30-06 bullet with a 270-caliber bullet! Another source of mercury contamination is often found in fish. Eating too much fish can cause problems. The high level of mercury in the water is usually due to natural sources of mercury. However, in some instances, high levels have resulted from contamination with mercury used in gold mining or from waste products being dumped into our lakes and streams from chemical plants.

Most doctors do not even consider the possibility of a toxic metal reaction, so unfortunately it is often overlooked and not tested for. Specific metal testing can be done with blood tests; however, I prefer hair analysis. It is less expensive and tends to measure tissue stores of the metal that are often greater than the serum level. There are so many causative factors that are polluting our environment with toxic metals that all of us are probably being exposed to some degree.
I recently became upset when I learned that in at least thirteen states they are mixing toxic chemicals with liquid fertilizers and are spraying them on the soils that produce the crops we consume! Earlier, I mentioned how vitamins, minerals and amino acid deficiencies can cause emotional and psychological disturbances. Well, so can toxic metal loads. Some mass murderers have been found to have high levels of manganese in their brain, which very well could have been responsible for their abnormal behavior.

Be aware that heavy metal poisoning is common and can occur not only from mercury and lead but also from elevated levels of phosphorus, copper, tin, cadmium, manganese, arsenic, aluminum, and so forth. These levels if elevated in the body can often be reduced by various chelating methods. Heavy metal poisoning is becoming more common. It can cause not only physical problems, but also emotional and neurological symptoms. Elevated lead levels are found in heavy smokers. Vitamin C, in 1000-2000 milligrams per day, has been found to lower the lead levels in smokers by over seventy-five percent.

As a general rule, I advise my patients not to have root canals. I've seen far too many patients with post-root-canal problems, both acute and chronic. If the dentist takes the time to do a good job and uses the proper sterile methods, the tooth root canals will not be a problem later.

There is much information on both mercury and root canals, so check with your local library or online computer. An excellent book, *Toxic Metal Syndrome,* discusses all the toxic metals in our environment and the health problems they can cause. You will be amazed and probably upset when you read this.

Two months ago, a patient from New Mexico came in. He was in a wheelchair and couldn't walk. He was diagnosed with Multiple Sclerosis. Kinesiology did not confirm the diagnosis of MS but did identify the probability of mercury toxicity and systemic Candida. He was started on mercury detox and ADP, which is an oregano extract. One month later at a follow-up visit he walked in using only a cane part-time! He has a way to go, but he is definitely grateful for his progress and has subsequently referred a number of new patients to me.

Chapter 7

Health Care Legislation

As this book is being written, House bill HR 745/S578, "Access to Medical Treatment Act," has not passed. By the time you read this, I pray it is the law of the land. If not, it is essential that you demonstrate your support for this critical piece of legislation by calling and writing your Congressman. Without HR 745/S578, your health options are in the hands of the federal bureaucrats. Since July 1, 1998, Medicare patients treated by a Medicare participating physician have not been able to obtain non-authorized alternative services, even if they are willing to pay for them out of their own pocket. To do so, you must see a physician who does not accept Medicare.

This bill also makes available safe, proven therapies that are not yet approved here by the FDA. Do you think our pharmaceutical industry might have some say in this? There is no economic incentive to spend years and millions of dollars to develop a natural non-patentable medication. Again, I use the example of the inexpensive "Black Ointment." It's cheap and it works, but who can afford the time and money to get it approved by the FDA? Our system just doesn't work that way.

The bill has many patient safeguards built into it to prevent quackery regarding medications and therapies. They must be safe and effective. Patients must see an authorized physician and be fully informed before receiving any therapy approved under this bill.

In order to provide my patients with treatment alternatives such as chelation, I had to opt out of Medicare, with a resultant loss of some patients. However, I believe that one must adhere to their principles regardless of the consequences. "Take a stand and make a mark!" House bill HR 745/S578 ensures the doctor-patient relationship. Patients have the right and ability to get the information they need to make an informed decision on their health care.

There is a new bill that you should contact your Senators about. The bill is S722 and it gives the FDA the power to take any supplement off the market at its sole discretion! All they need is to have one single complaint about the product. Evidence that it is harmful is not required. Contrast that to prescription drugs.

They must have a large number of serious side effects and kill more than one individual before the FDA will consider taking them off the market.

Previously L-tryptophane was banned when a few batches were contaminated and harmed some people. It was proved that the contamination and not the L-trytophane was the problem. Yet the FDA took it off the market and we still do not have access to this extremely beneficial amino acid.

After what you have read in my book plus what you already know about nutritional therapy, it is very important that you do your utmost to defeat this unjust Senate Bill 722.

So call your Senators *now* and e-mail them at http://capwiz.com via a simple Web form. Scroll down to "Action Alert" and click under Support S1538 and oppose S722.

Thank you. Your support is urgently needed. Your health is at stake.

Chapter 8

Stroke of Luck

I was in the process of preparing this book for publication in September, 2001. My first wife, Shirlee, had been battling lung cancer for over one year. She finally became terminal and was hospitalized in Springerville, Arizona. My current wife, Kathy, and I drove to Springerville and rented a motel room. I spent a week, day and night with Shirlee and the children, mostly for the children's support. At the end of the week Shirlee left this earth and I returned home to my practice for several days. One week later I returned to St. John, Arizona, for her funeral and stayed an extra day at my daughter's home. I returned home Sunday afternoon and on Monday, October 1, I woke up and realized that something was wrong. My left side felt unusual; I thought I had slept on it wrong. But then when I got into the kitchen I couldn't hold anything and dropped my favorite coffee cup on the floor and it broke. The phone rang and I had trouble talking. Only then did I realize I had had a stroke. I went into the bathroom and looked into the mirror and saw the left side of my face all distorted. I was able to take a shower then went into the bedroom. I woke my wife and told her I had some bad news. I then told her I had had a stroke and was going to the office to get some treatment. She was alarmed and told me she would drive me to the office even though I felt I could do it—after all, my right side was OK! Upon arriving at the office, I found that my blood pressure was very high 240/120. Obviously, with Shirlee's illness I had not been taking care of myself and watching my pressure even though I was on blood pressure medication.

I was surprised that the stroke did not cause me any concern or worry whatsoever. I figured my wife would do enough worrying for us both and she did. I felt comfortable in relying on my alternative medicine knowledge. I promptly started an intravenous EDTH chelation treatment. My nurse, office manager and wife all ganged up on me and insisted that I see my cardiologist, Dr. Risk, who is an excellent physician even though he practices traditional medicine. He admitted me to the hospital for two days to take the standard X-rays and CAT scans. Dr. George Brian also examined me in neurological consultation. As I was getting ready to leave the hospital, a chest X-ray was ordered. Why, I don't know, but this is where my "stroke of luck" occurred. The X-ray revealed my trachea to be deviated considerably to the right, without the cause being obvious. Therefore, a CAT scan was ordered that I had to return to the hospital to obtain. The scan report revealed a large aneurysm on the ascending aorta next to the heart and in the proximal segment of the aortic arch. This is a very unusual site. I had never seen one in this area in my forty-two years of practice; however, one of my medical school classmates had a similar problem two years prior.

My brother had an abdominal aortic aneurysm two years before, so it may be a hereditary factor as both my brother and I also have hypertension and diabetes. Instead of being upset that it had been found, I was very grateful and thanked God that it had been found in time for repair as there had not been any symptoms. I truly believe that my stroke had been one of luck as the aneurysm would probably not have been found in time.

Following the stroke, my only concern was whether I had lost my intuitive abilities. A patient was brought into the next bed of my hospital room. From behind the curtain I thought about him for a few seconds and then told my wife what I had interpreted. The next day I was able to talk with the gentleman and substantiated that my diagnosis of him had been correct. I then quit worrying. My intuitive ability had been retained.

Thanks to intravenous chelation with EDTA that I took on a daily and then every other day basis, I recovered from my stroke very quickly and was able to return to work half days after only one week, much to the surprise of my physicians! My facial weakness cleared mostly after one month. I have seen chelation therapy work wonders for every stroke patient I have treated. I feel strongly that every stroke patient should be given a choice of a treatment of intravenous chelation with EDTA.

In February 2002, I traveled to Houston, Texas, to have my aneurysm repaired by Dr. Cocilli. I was referred to him by Dr. Ted Ditrick, head of the Arizona Heart Institute and also by a vascular surgeon in Tucson, for whom my daughter has worked. I don't think I could have been referred to anyone better. My operation was February 7, and I don't have much memory of the next ten days. I do remember that the day after surgery I told Laurie "Happy Birthday." I hadn't forgotten. Barbie, a very good friend, recently told me something that I had forgotten. She had talked with me following surgery and I had told her that during the surgery I had "seen the light." I'm sorry I don't have any recollection of that event.

It has taken the muscles longer to recover than I had anticipated; however, my classmate who had the same surgery keeps telling me that this is not unusual and also to expect to be depressed. Luckily my depression was very mild and required no medication. My main concern was the persistent exhaustion that kept me from returning to work. I finally decided to return two mornings a week in July.

Thankfully, in mid-June, a nutritionist who is a good friend and patient suggested that I try soluble rice bran. I was amazed that within a week my energy improved and I felt like returning to work. It has been two months since I started the soluble rice bran product, and I am rapidly regaining my former stamina and abilities. Very much to my surprise, I have been able to reduce my blood pressure pills from four to one a day. Here's another big plus for alternative therapy, in my estimation. In the past six weeks I have also employed two other alternative therapies, with excellent results. I healed three abscesses under my arm with Transfer Factor Plus instead of antibiotics. I also removed two lesions from my face that were very suspicious for melanoma with the black herbal ointment I discussed in an earlier chapter.

So as you can see, I not only advise but actually use the products and endorse what I have written about.

To recap, I want to state again several things that I feel need to be repeated.

- Everyone, especially health care professionals, need to learn and use kinesiology. It is the intelligent way to determine what and how many supplements you need to stay healthy.

- Intravenous chelation should be one of your first choices when preventing or treating a heart attack or stroke.

- Intravenous hydrogen peroxide can be a life saver when used to treat serious infections—especially—viral and also is very helpful for many other conditions, including emphysema.

- Collosonia Root is excellent for the treatment of hemorrhoids.

- Don't forget to overcome your aversions and try urine therapy.

- A simple and inexpensive therapy for toenail fungus is Vicks VapoRub applied twice a day or daily urine soaks.

- If you smash a fingernail and get a very painful bleeding under the nail, it can be quickly relieved by heating a paper clip red hot and just touching the nail.

- It's good to remember the use of cayenne pepper to stop bleeding both internal and external. Just mix a tablespoon with a glass of water and drink it as needed or apply locally for external wounds.

- A hot shower and breathing the hot, humid air will improve many acute respiratory problems.

- A temperature of up to 102 is not harmful and doesn't need to be treated. It's just a good sign that the body's defenses are working against an infection.

- There are many nutritional supplements to help improve our immune system and to correct many of our chronic conditions. Again, it is very important to use kinesiology to determine the best ones for you. Remember, everyone is different and what is good for the goose is not always good for the gander!

- Foot massage can be a very effective first line of medical management. I have effectively treated everything from headache to angina with it. Simply massage the sole of each foot until you find a tender area and then slowly massage each area until the symptom improves.

- Don't drink tap water if at all possible.

- Homocystein and c-reactive protein levels are much more important than cholesterol levels.

- Don't be afraid of eating red meat and eggs. They are both very good for you, if you are not allergic to them.

- Eat a large percentage of your daily diet *raw*. Cooking destroys enzymes that are very beneficial to you. Choose vegetables with many different colors.

- Neonatal glandular supplements have been found to be very effective in strengthening specific organ functions, such as heart, adrenal, pituitary, and so on.

- To date, the group of biological compounds that have shown the greatest protection from aging are the antioxidants. There are many antioxidants and we have found that the more we take in number, not necessarily in amount, the more effective they seem to be.

- Two foods that we have been told to avoid—salt and coffee—can now be viewed in a different light. I still believe that commercial salt that has been adulterated is not good; however, natural sea salt with all its inherent ingredients is safe in small to moderate amounts. Check the label carefully. Make sure it has not been heated or had chemicals added. Recently it has been shown that coffee and caffeine in limited amounts are probably OK. Time and more research will tell us the answer.

- Sunshine does not cause an increase of skin cancer, although frequent *sunburns* may predispose you to developing it. I believe that a good suntan (natural) is very good for you.

- Don't forget the possibility of allergy—food, chemicals, materials, and so forth, can cause any symptoms you can possible think of.

- Give everyone a big hug and love your neighbor. Love and forgive everyone and do not judge.

Chapter 9

Reflections

The best way to survive an uncertain future is with prevention and preparation. Throughout this book I have stressed the importance of strengthening our immune systems. This is critical. Why do some people in a household get sick while other members do not? They have all undoubtedly been exposed to the same infectious agents. The difference is their immune defenses. I like to use the illustration of a yard surrounded by a picket fence, with many dogs outside the fence. All it takes is for one or two pickets to be removed and the dogs come in, just as the infectious agents can invade your body if your immune defense is defective.

Unfortunately, improving your immune system will be more difficult in the future. The United Nations is doing its best to control the availability of natural medications, even in the United States. The FDA purposely limits the development, testing and manufacture of new medicines. These are attacks on our individual freedoms. We must take a stand against the government's efforts to take away our access to any and all health care.

I have tried to bridge the two worlds of medicine, traditional (allopathic) and alternative (integrated.) The attention of the open-minded health care provider must be on wellness and not solely on treatment. One of the reasons I moved to Arizona was to associate with medical doctors of like mind. I became a member of the Arizona Homeopathic Integrative Medical Association, which is the best of its kind in the United States. This organization is composed of M.D.'s, D.O.'s, Dentists, Chiropractors, Homeopaths and doctors in allied fields. All members believe and practice alternative integrated medicine.

I have heard of doctors who don't believe a physician can practice alternative medicine and allopathic medicine at the same time. However, I can assure you that it can and is being done. I am particularly happy knowing that the concept of alternative medicine is growing among allopathic physicians. Dr. Andrew Weil of Tucson, Arizona has opened a clinic in association with the University of Arizona. Residents are taught how integrative medicine works in practice. To my knowledge, it is the only program of its kind to offer such training for physicians. There are, however, other centers where alternative medicine is practiced and evaluated under the auspices of the Office of Alternative Medicine (OAM) of the National Institutes of Health. These centers are located at Stanford University, Columbia University and the Universities of Texas, California and Maryland.

Many patients who use alternative methods never mention this to their physicians for fear of ridicule and rejection. In many instances they feel more knowledgeable about the alternative treatment than their physician. Patients need to discuss and even enlighten their physicians about a particular alternative therapy. I'm sure that this would help bridge the gap in treatment philosophies. Also, I strongly believe that the patients' demand for alternative therapies will increase their availability. More and more patients are opposed to using chemical prescription medications that tend to suppress their symptoms without treating the cause of the problem.

Take prescription medication when necessary. When you don't need it, get off it! If the side effects are worse than what you are being treated for, use your common sense and explore a different option. It is not wise to stop any prescription medication without first discussing this with your doctor! For serious conditions it is wise to get another medical opinion. Often, you will find that there are more conservative treatments available.

Our world is changing. Major problems will continue to plague us in the future: governmental and economic instability, wars, violence in our streets, terrorism, a shortage of fresh food and water, abnormal manmade weather conditions and earth changes. Drug-resistant infections, toxic waste, alcohol and drug abuse. These and perhaps worse problems will cause tremendous personal stress. *Women's Health Magazine* had some suggestions for coping with this stress.

- Laughter is often the best remedy. Find a reason to laugh.

- Enjoy the people in your life who make you happy and allow yourself time with them.

- Don't waste your time by reliving mistakes. Mistakes are to learn from, not to rehash.

- Learn to recognize what you can control and let go of what you can't. I would add three more suggestions:

- Love everyone even if you might not like them. This is the key to healthy living.

- Abide by the Golden Rule in all you do.
- Own gold and silver.

Life is hard by the yard,

But by the inch,

It's a cinch.

Postscript

I couldn't let this book go to print without bringing you up to date on my problems with "Big Brother" (the Arizona State Medical Board). I have commented on our relationship in a previous chapter. They let me alone for several years but are now again causing me problems. It is not just Arizona State—it is also Federal. In 1998 a law was passed that prohibited a physician who practiced alternative medicine to be a Medicare participant, so I had to let go of all my Medicare patients except those who wanted to continue under my care and pay cash for their visits.

It was recently brought to my attention again that the "quack busters" are at it again and your health freedom is seriously threatened!

It stems from a meeting of the Federation of State Medical Boards several years ago where a concerted effort was announced (and recorded) to systematically revoke the licenses of all complementary and alternative doctors in the country, state by state. They also intended to repeal laws already passed in several states that protected basic human medical rights.

In North Carolina, which followed Alaska in protecting your rights, the medical board has decided to ignore the protective provisions in the law completely and has adopted a policy to go after every integrative physician in the state, even with the law on the books!

In Wisconsin, the medical board has publicly acknowledged that it intends to get rid of every doctor in the state who veers from pushing chemical medicine. Doctors who use nutritional supplements instead of drugs will be smoked out and rubbed out. If they prevail in Wisconsin, all states are at risk. The multinational pharmaceutical companies are losing money and are very concerned about more losses due to patients preferring natural therapies. The allopathic medical societies are also very concerned about the monetary aspect, since patients are spending millions of dollars for alternative care.

Please contact your state attorney general and demand that he or she order your medical board to cease exterminating alternative physicians and demand implementation of policies that will forever protect your decisions in the privacy of your physician's office. Very recently I have been placed on probation, prohibiting me from practicing alternative medicine at the same time that I practice standard allo-pathic medicine. My case was heard by an Administrative Law Judge, David G. Martin. He disagreed with me that I could pick and choose which medical "hat" I would wear (homeopathic versus allopathic) while engaging in the practice of med-icine. In other words, I am now forbidden to evaluate, diagnose, and prescribe what I think best for a patient based on my comprehensive knowledge of both standard medicine and alternative medicine. I do not know how I can refraim: it would be like trying to live without breathing. I have several options and at this date have not decided which to pursue. One, give up my allopathic license and practice solely under my homeopathic license. Two, continue to fight for my rights. I asked for a hearing on this decision and was granted a ten-minute hearing only. Unfortunately I could not find this new location in a timely manner (I was four minutes late) and I was refused the opportunity to present my case. I have asked for a rehearing but that has been refused also.

My patients cannot believe that this decision by the Administrative Court and Arizona Board of Medicine has any merit, nor do I. Unfortunately, at the pres-ent time I do not have adequate funds to pursue this further legally.

January 04 Update

The Arizona Board of Medicine has continued to harrass me for use of alternate methods of healing—particularly chelation. As a result, I surrendered my med-ical license in Arizona on December 30, 2003. I now practice under my Arizona homeopathic license that allows me to practice as I please using all options avail-able to me. I will probably also surrender my New Mexico license next year as I feel I no longer need it.

Testimonials

My friend asked me to write a few words for his book. There's so much I'd like to say about the most caring, kind, loving, non-judgmental individual I have had the pleasure and honor to call my doctor, and next to my wife, my best friend.

I met Dr. Gene Schroeder thirty years ago and over the years I've slowly had the good fortune to get closer to him.

I will now take this opportunity to just say thank you for your friendship and love and also for saving my life the natural way with chelation therapy instead of bypass surgery.

Above all…thank you for being my friend.

P.S. It would take another book to list every "natural" cure you've helped me and my family with!

A friend you can never be rid of
H. G. "Bob" Artibee
Negaunee, Michigan

Dear Dr. Schroeder,

I want to thank you for helping my wife with her medical condition and controlling her high blood pressure. She feels a lot better. Thank you also for helping me with my health. Doc, on a scale of one to ten, I would have to rate you over a ten. I thank God I really found a doctor that not only knows what he is doing, but also a caring doctor. I might add, you are more than fair for what you charge; to think I have spent all my money on doctors that not only over-charge me but did not know what they were doing. I don't know where they got their training.

Well, doctor, thanks again and God bless you.

Sincerely,
Frank and Irene Celona
Prescott, Arizona

August 1998 was special for me because that is when I first met Dr. Gene Schroeder. I'd heard a little about how he diagnosed through the use of kinesiology and felt it would be great to have my allergies individualized.

Feeling like my body didn't know what to do with food, was frustrating. When Dr. Schroeder expressed the very same thought to me, I was elated. Finally, a doctor who could tell me what was wrong! Following his advice for two months brought my triglycerides down over 502 points. Suddenly I was becoming better. All my problems dropped into the normal range. No more cardiac risk! Wow! Praise to God and thanks to Dr. Schroeder for sharing his gift.

> Betty Carroll
> Prescott, Arizona

It is with great pleasure that I speak a few words regarding Dr. Gene Schroeder and his methods of practicing medicine. Because it would take lengthy pages to adequately describe the love and compassion I've seen this truly dedicated physician demonstrate while administering to his fellow human beings—both patients and nonpatients. I would like to say this: To those of you who have read "Henri and the Angels," a main character referred to as Dr. Gene depicts exactly the true character of Dr. Gene Schroeder of whom I now speak.

I have since written my 'memoirs' where I tell about my life and involvements with my Guardian Angel named James. Entitled 'Coping', my memoirs tell of how James insists I remain on a healthy diet and follow only the expert advice of Dr. Gene Schroeder.

Because of Dr. Gene's methods of healing, at age fifty-five I remain healthy and disease-free.

> Ellen St. James, Co-author
> "Henri and the Angels"
> Quinn, Michigan

I first heard of Dr. Schroeder about three years ago, when my physical and emotional well-being were at odds and sleep was difficult to come by. Months later, during a horrible, restless night, his name kept flashing through my mind. It was then that I decided to seek his medical advice. So, for the past two and one half years, I have been seeing him about every three months.

With his amazing intuition and kinesiology skills, my physical and emotional well-being have greatly improved, not by medication and expensive diagnostic tests, but by dietary supplements appropriate to meet my body's needs and requirements. As a result of this treatment, my arteries are freer from build-up (arteriosclerosis), my bone density has increased, my cholesterol level has dropped fifty points and my blood pH is now neutral, resulting in far less tartar or plaque build-up and healthier gums. My energy level has increased, allowing me to engage in activities that at the age of seventy-five are denied many people. He has made it possible for me to live everyday to the fullest. He is a compassionate, caring person. No matter how busy his day, he always has time to care for your needs, engage in friendly conversation and end the visit with a hug.

Mary Anderson
Prescott, Arizona

Finding a medical doctor like "Doctor Gene" (as we call him) in this small city was a pleasant surprise. He is versed in most alternative methods as his book shows. We're an eighty-two year-old couple who adhere to natural ways and have since our youth. In large cities we used to call home, we never found a doctor like him. As his book shows, he has had an extensive education in many disciplines, including surgery. Now he concentrates on keeping his patients well, as his "Wellness Clinic" suggests. We feel fortunate to have found him to help us stay well.

Sincerely,
Mary & Don Briggs
Prescott, Arizona

We are all on a journey through life, leaving our footprints on the sands of time. Dr. Schroeder's journey combines traditional medicine with alternative methods.

In thought field therapy he taps the healing spirit within us by eliminating negative thought patterns, which allows us to source our inner healing powers.

Amazing results! Great message and dedication to healing.

Jim & Evelyn Phelan
Prescott, Arizona

My first visit to Dr. Schroeder was for nutritional advice. At first, I was doubtful of his use of kinesiology but over the past two years and after several visits, I find he has usually been correct in helping me identify foods and supplements that either agree or disagree with me as an individual. He particularly stresses that each patient is an individual and that no single mold fits everyone.

He has been of help to me in other ways as well. For instance, he has spotted potential medical problems before they have manifested themselves and instituted methods to prevent them from becoming real problems. He also has been quick to suggest any other treatment or procedure in which conventional or technical medical practice is needed and for which I would need to go elsewhere for such treatment.

Roland Hellin
Prescott, Arizona

I have known Dr. Schroeder for the past ten years. He provided me with a thorough medical evaluation after a urologist recommended surgery for prostate cancer. Dr. Schroeder helped me explore various treatment options. I value his extensive knowledge and experience with surgery, with nutrition, with spiritual sensitivity, with alternative healing resources and his desire to enter into a collaborative relationship with me. I trust him and his use of multiple skills, though I feel I could differ with him and continue to work with him. I value his concern for life, and not just physical life. Therefore, I have no hesitation in recommending Dr. Schroeder as a dedicated physician.

The Rev. Paul W. Strickland
Prescott Valley, Arizona

I can't tell you how many traditional doctors I've seen in the last ten years here in Prescott and Prescott Valley and how much money I've spent on useless drugs which did me no good. I still had problems with aches, pains, sinus problems and just about everything else. My friend told me about Dr. Schroeder, and after one visit I was completely sold on this doctor. I felt he really cared about me and listened to what I was saying. His diagnoses and medications worked every time. Dr. Gene is an extremely intuitive physician who knows how to integrate traditional with alternative therapies for our benefit. Many thanks to Dr. Schroeder, kinesiology, and thought field therapy, and so on and so forth.

Jan Boylan
Prescott Valley, Arizona

I have been a patient of Dr. Gene Schroeder for the past nine years, as has my husband.

I started seeing him for tennis elbow due to excessive computer work. With natural supplements and traditional medicines, we have gotten it under control—which was much better than under the knife.

The key to our doctor/patient relationship has been his attempt at always trying natural healing as well as modern-day medicine.

Through the years I've been through highs and lows, like any "active" person. Dr. Gene has always been there to listen, express an opinion and most importantly, offer a hug! I have always felt a sort of kinship toward him; nothing shocks him, and he's a very down to earth, loving, caring man. Over the years I've come to also know Dr. Gene's wife, Kathy, who in her own right is a very neat person. You know the saying: behind every successful man, there's a great woman.

What always clues me in on a doctor's true being is how his office staff behaves. I've always been treated with the utmost respect and they always seem to really enjoy their job and working along with Dr. Gene.

I have referred many people over the years to Dr. Schroeder. Not a one has come away without feeling that they had, finally, really been listened to and helped.

I am a forty-two year-old female who has had my share of female "stuff." Dr. Gene is the only doctor that I've encountered that truly listens…Doesn't that say it all???

> Sincerely,
> Diane M. Baccus
> Prescott, Arizona

Dr. Schroeder provides a medical model for me, blending allopathic and complementary medicine in a gentle and respectful way. He treats me as an individual, recognizing that two people with the same symptoms may have different problems and may require different treatment. His diagnostic abilities are revolutionary, using the response from my body and his own experience, knowledge and intuition to accurately diagnose problems that would require expensive testing to properly diagnose in the allopathic method and in some cases would be impossible to recognize. He uses the same approach in treating conditions, asking my body what would work best for me whether that be the use of supplements, herbs, essential oils, homeopathy, thought field therapy, allopathic medicine or some other treatment with which he is familiar. He has been an incredible support and a facilitator of my healing process, allowing me to heal in an efficient and non-invasive manner. I am so grateful for his help and his willingness to risk working outside mainstream medicine in order to help people in a way that is consistent with his own integrity.

Janet A. Eichorst
Prescott, Arizona

Dr. Gene Schroeder has brought me through numerous crises. I have food allergies that change from time to time and give me a variety of symptoms, from mild to horrendous. Along with allergies, I have a heart problem that varies from atypical beats to atrial fibrillation. Trust and caring are the cornerstones of my relationship with him. His broad-based knowledge gives me the confidence that he is right in his treatment program for me. Even when I can't figure out how it could work, and I don't exactly follow his order, I later have to admit, "Well, I guess he was right!" His follow-up phone calls to "see how I'm doing" are comforting and reassuring.

Martha C. Strickland
Prescott Valley, Arizona

For years I suffered from debilitating heart palpitations with dizziness. I sought treatment from a nationally known clinic and was diagnosed with a heart disease. It was highly recommended that I get a pacemaker and start on heart medication. Instead, I chose to see an alternative doctor and sought out Dr. Schroeder.

Dr. Schroeder, using a form of kinesiology called CRA, diagnosed a thyroid problem and suggested a natural form of thyroid medication. With the medication, the palpitations have drastically improved and I have been relatively symptom-free for five years.

I think Dr. Schroeder is a visionary and an extremely intuitive physician who has a gift for integrating traditional and complementary medicine.

Dr. Elaine A. Hodge,
Licensed Psychologist
Director, Holistic Psychological
Association
Marquette, Michigan

My first meeting with Dr. Gene Schroeder was through an appointment made by an insurance company.

I was so impressed with his knowledge and thoroughness that a decision was made immediately. He was the person I wanted to continue monitoring my health.

A patient is the beneficiary of this unusual doctor's gifts including kinesiology with homeopathy.

Anne Gillow
Prescott, Arizona

Having suffered from candidiasis for ten years with no relief or progress in sight, I met Dr. Schroeder, who had no difficulty in treating my symptoms with nutritional remedies with great success. Today I'm enjoying excellent health.

Ernie Freddy Campbell
Prescott, Arizona

After using cortisone, due to Addisons disease for thirty-two years, it became ineffective and started causing other physical symptoms. Dr. Schroeder supervised my withdrawal from cortisone, substituting some nutritional medicines. Thanks to his expertise in the medical and homeopathic fields, I am free of drugs and healthier than I have ever been.

Jacquelyn West Campbell
Prescott Valley, Arizona

We have been patients of Dr. Schroeder for several years and truly appreciate his integrity and holistic approach. He has the rare quality of listening to you, and incorporating all methods for your total well being.

Melvin and Darleen Johansen
Prescott, Arizona

Dr. Schroeder is a very unique doctor. He has all of the obvious medical degrees and he possesses something far more important—he is what I call a medically intuitive doctor, able to read things in the body that are now always obvious.

During my first visit to him, I was in his office only a few minutes when he announced that I had a blockage in the right side of my colon, blocked with medication build-up. He recommended colonics, which I did six months later. The series of colonics shocked the therapist with how much medication build-up passed. The pain was gone in my lower right side for good. Dr. Schroeder's large variety of skills have helped me heal at a much more rapid speed and I have saved a fortune on unnecessary tests. He is a real Godsend!

Carol Rutherford
Prescott, Arizona

Prior to starting medical care with Dr. Schroeder, my experience with most doctors was frustrating, expensive, and patronizing. Finding Dr. Schroeder was like finding treasure. He listens to me and believes me. He makes me feel safe and comfortable, so I know I am in good, competent hands. This is a far cry from the assorted MDs and specialists I was seeing for over ten years. They either could not, or would not, help me.

By contrast, Dr. Gene exhibits the knowledge and creativity to see between seemingly unrelated symptoms, and he has the ability to adapt treatments that quickly heal the source of the problem. He puts the patient's individualized tests and remedies into a comprehensive program that starts working with your first visit.

Dr. Gene is a healer who is kind and competent. He has true courage, ethics, skill and dedication to his patient, and he helps his profession to evolve. He does not let bureaucracy stop him; he keeps learning and developing his intuition and versatility.

Currently, all my symptoms and syndromes are accounted for and are being treated effectively. At long last, I am beginning to have periods of sustained improvement. I have fewer acute or serious relapses and exacerbations, even though they do occur. So it is a great relief to know that my doctor is available for speedy assistance.

Now I understand why I was guided into an unplanned and sudden move from California to Prescott. The doctor I really needed, Dr. Gene Schroeder, M.D. is here. I am, indeed, thankful that he is.

Kathleen Magique, RM. DC.
Retired
Prescott, Arizona

Having succumbed to the general marketing fervor that pervades the health food industry, I was taking over fifty supplemental vitamins, herbs, minerals, and tinctures each day. My over-supplementing was fueled both by desire to get enough of the right stuff, and by the fear that I might be missing something. Dr. Gene Schroeder evaluated my condition and my supplement habits. He discovered that, for my particular individual constitution, ninety percent of the health food trends to which I was subjecting myself were not only unnecessary, but were actually fatiguing me as my body processed them. I now take a multiple vitamin, C, E, and thyroid. I feel healthy, balanced, and "free at last" from the health food industry hype marketing campaigns.

Robert Rutherford
Prescott, Arizona

Dr. Gene Schroeder was my lifesaver. God has truly given him a gift to help the sick. I am a forty year-old woman that started having terrible pains (worse than childbirth) in my stomach. After three trips to the ER and six different doctors' opinions and seven months of throwing up green bile, blood test after blood test, and thousands of dollars later, my husband made an appointment with Dr. Gene. Within thirty minutes he told me exactly what was wrong with me (gallstones)—even down to the size. I love and believe in him and his staff. Thanks, Dr. Gene.

Paula Faith Slaughter
Humboldt, Arizona

I am a forty-two year-old male going through life with chronic back pain. I am being treated by Dr. Gene with the right pain management that works for me. I have been to many doctors and none of them are as understanding as Dr. Gene. I can talk to him as a friend as well as a doctor. There is a family atmosphere with him and his staff. If I'm going through a hard time, I can call him up and talk to him on the phone and he always makes me feel better. More doctors should be like Dr. Gene Schroeder! Thank you Dr. Gene for your kindness, understanding, and helping me get through my pain.

God bless you, your family, and your staff.

With loving regards,
Guy Slaughter & Family
Humboldt, Arizona

Dr. Schroeder is my physician of many years, and I am health-conscious. It is wonderful and beneficial to have a doctor that knows alternative medicine besides being a medical doctor. I feel Dr. Schroeder is very knowledgeable in his kinesiology and homeopathic/holistic fields.

He has always been a very caring person that takes pride in his patient's wellbeing, and never minded us calling him at odd hours if we needed him.

His sensitivity to his medicine, whether it is holistic or orthodox, makes him a great doctor that can give us an accurate diagnosis.

> Cecilia Hawkins
> Skull Valley, Arizona

My brother-in-law, in Michigan, called in desperation with a bad case of shingles that needed to be cleared up fast so that he could leave in a few days for a very important overseas business trip. I told him to call Dr. Gene. After jokingly saying "Isn't that your witch doctor?" he reluctantly made the phone call. Before he told Dr. Gene his problem, my intuitive doctor told him what was wrong and how to get rid of it. This brother-in-law was astounded. Doubtful because he hadn't "doctored" in this sort of way, he visited an alternative doctor in his area. A second opinion turned out to be the exact treatment Dr. Gene had advised.

My brother-in-law called me wanting me to call Gene and tell him thanks for the quick cure. Laughing, he said he didn't want to call because Gene might find something else wrong with him.

> Bill Calkins
> Grand Rapids, Michigan

Dr. Schroeder has been my doctor for the past nine years. He has been the most caring and thorough doctor I've ever had. Treating me with kinesiology I feel saves me lots of money on tests and I only take the amount I need of vitamins or prescriptions. I feel more like a twenty year-old than a sixty-one year-old.

> Ann Daly
> Paulden, Arizona

Dr. Schroeder is a health care provider who listens and knows that good health is achieved through a balance of mind, body and spirit. Through his unique and oh so accurate testing, I am finally being treated with medications that enhance rather than poison my health.

Thank you, Dr. Schroeder, for you are truly gifted!

Cora Bailey
Reno, Nevada

We met Dr. Gene in January 1988 and even having moved apart 2,000 miles, we still return for his care and advice only, as all other doctors have failed in "attempt" or treatment and constant care of myself and family. He's never failed us or let us down like most other physicians we encountered! On two occasions I've been told the following, by other physicians or "peers" (he has none). I was first told about 10 years ago "That's the most caring and intelligent man I've ever spoken to. Never lose him!" Then as recently as one year ago I was told "That's not a doctor! That's a saint."

Quite possibly, at any rate always our family friend and physician as long as he has his practice and I practice life.

All our thanks, respect, and
far more, love
The Heinzeroth's
Rockford, Illinois

Although my wife has been a patient and ardent supporter of Dr. Schroeder for several years, I was very skeptical of her reports of his methods of diagnosis and treatment.

A persistent and painful ailment from which I suffered returned and did not respond to the antibiotics previously prescribed by doctors over the years. In desperation, I visited Dr. Schroeder. In one visit, he correctly diagnosed the problem and prescribed a combination herbal and vitamin ritual. Within two weeks I was totally cured, and the problem has not reoccurred.

I became an immediate convert, and for the past few years, I have been a healthy and totally satisfied patient of Dr. Schroeder.

David R. Porter
Prescott, Arizona

I have been a patient of Dr. Gene Schroeder for approximately eight years. Being a doctor's daughter, I experienced from my father the best of care and from other doctors, adequate to less than adequate regard.

For several years I had a rapid weight gain and infections. The various physicians were doubtful I was truthful about my records showing the amount of food I was consuming, and prescribed various antibiotics for the infections. I was totally discouraged by the time I sat in Dr. Schroeder's office. Immediately he sensed my apprehension and despair, and he responded to me with sensitivity and professionalism.

He ordered the blood tests that I had taken before, but most important, he tested me with kinesiology. He treated me for a low thyroid and with vitamin herb therapy for the other physical problems that had developed. Suffice it to say, at all times Dr. Schroeder has been accurate, successful, caring and supportive throughout the years. In him I have well-earned total confidence.

Kaye M. Porter
Prescott, Arizona

How best to describe Dr. Gene Schroeder? Words are almost impossible to describe his work and dedication to his patients and the medical profession. He has never failed me for he has always been there for me whether it be night or day when I needed him most. I can say, "I can always count on Dr. Gene." I suffer from spinal disease and its other friends and medical maladies: fibromyalgia, neck pain, chronic back pain, and a parade of illness that goes on. All this because of a careless driver. Some of America's best doctors said, "Nothing could be done for me and that includes a Dean from "Harvard Medical School," who was the Chief Fellow in endocrinology who did not even recognize the signs and symptoms that I have hypo-thyroidism, yet Dr. Gene did. Yes, even Harvard said, "Why don't you apply for disability, we will be more than happy to sign the papers." I said, "I need a life and to work; that's more important to me than anything."

They did not care or believe that I could overcome my medical problems or ever work again. When I met Dr. Gene he believed in me and knew instinctively that I spoke the truth. In a short time I had to have triple C-Spine Fusion five, six, and seven. This eliminated a lot of my pain but not all of it. Most important to me was that he kept me from being paralyzed and more important, he kept working and he gave me my life back and prevented me from needing welfare and applying for disability. For I have regained my dignity in the "Professional

Community" and the working community at large and now I'm on the mend. I could say much more in the behalf of Dr. Gene Schroeder for it goes on and on in praise for Dr. Gene and they would be endless.

Kimberly Williams, R. E.

Gene is one of the most caring and thoughtful persons that I have ever had the pleasure of working with. He has always been on the "cutting edge" of alternative therapies, willing to go out on that proverbial limb to help his patient get well. He shares not only his knowledge but also his precious time with anyone who may have a question or who just needs to talk. I am proud to know him personally and professionally, and to call him my friend.

Jane A. Kohner
Prescott Valley, Arizona

During these past eleven years, I have been blessed by friendship and medical care from Dr. Gene and his lovely wife, Kathy. They both (and he in particular) have done for me what no other doctor has done. I thank God for their care and Gene's skills. He has been the only doctor, to date, who has accurately diagnosed my metabolic condition. To any other doctor who may read this, please, do not be afraid to learn.

Darwin L. Teos
Prescott, Arizona

W. G. Schroeder has not referred to himself as any of the now-popular genre of practitioners. He is not simply a faith healer, or a medical intuitive, nor is he a quack as the title suggests. He is a man, educated in medicine with the title "M.D." and has practiced throughout his lifetime without lapses of medical ethics and more importantly his own higher standards. He has consciously and super-consciously been on a life path of truth, love and knowledge. He has been endowed with teachers and angels who light his way. He has walked in a world of "healing" while others simply apply a band-aid for a dollar. He has been held in judgment, close scrutiny and the harsh criticism of "colleagues" with limited belief systems and field of vision and has not allowed their resistance to hamper his progress.

Dr. Schroeder has sought and received many of the spiritual gifts referred to in Corinthians (12:7-10). He is not a "Seer out of Season" as Cayce, who had no medical background, was dubbed. The "proof is in the pudding…" W. G. Schroeder's time is now.

D. Chaperon
Iron Mountain, Michigan

When I came to Dr. Schroeder's Rainbow Wellness Clinic in Prescott, Arizona, I was in a state of near death from congestive heart failure and circulatory problems. My condition was so critical that the good holistic physician, Dr. Schroeder, had grave doubts if he could save me. True to his kind and caring nature, he valiantly went all-out in trying to save my life!

His expertise in the healing arts is near miraculous. He took me from the dark shadow of approaching death to a bright world of blessed hope. I don't believe he has an equal in alternative therapy. Natural medicines work with the body, whereas conventional "cures" work against the body, as good Dr. Schroeder has so aptly demonstrated. Had I remained in Wisconsin under the incompetent health-destroying "care" of conventional physicians and their poisonous drugs, I would not be here today commending the brilliant non-conformist doctor of Prescott *who saved my life*, which brings up a final thought. "Who are the real quacks?"

In eternal gratitude,
Truman Smith
Bessie Babbet Wilderness Area
Florence, Wisconsin 54121

I was born in 1916 and am eighty-five years old.

In October 1999 I left the VA Hospital in a wheelchair with an oxygen tank by my side. My diagnosis was heart failure with blocked arteries and the VA gave me six months to live.

I spoke with my VA doctor and told her I was not going to die this way. I mentioned chelation treatment (which I read about), and her response was, "It is not medically proven effective." I was dismayed and left her office still needing oxygen.

I am a ballroom dance instructor at the local college along with my wife. On the way to school, I would use oxygen and at break time I would go out to the car and put my tank on for a few minutes. I proceeded to teach class and nobody knew of my dilemma.

By word of mouth, I heard more about chelation and found Dr. Schroeder. After five intravenous chelation treatments, I was off my oxygen, chest pain was gone and swelling in my legs was decreased tremendously.

Now, after twenty-three chelation treatments, I feel better, look younger and continue to teach dancing. People have guessed my age to be fifty-five or sixty.

I thank God for Dr. Schroeder and call him a saint. He is both intuitive and has a gift for healing. My sincere and heartfelt thanks to this great man.

Jivantoro
Prescott Valley, Arizona

About the Author

W. G. SCHROEDER, M.D., HMD

Gene Schroeder is founder of the Rainbow Wellness Clinic in Prescott, Arizona, where he has been practicing general, holistic, alternative, preventative and homeopathic medicine since 1996. He is licensed to practice medicine in Arizona and New Mexico and has been previously licensed in Wisconsin, North Dakota, Alaska and Michigan.

Gene's conventional medical education began in 1960 when he graduated from the University of Michigan Medical School. After completing a rotating internship at Borgess Hospital in Kalamazoo, Michigan, Gene joined a group practice in Ishpeming, Michigan from 1961 to 1966 that included general surgery. His foray into alternative medicine began while he was serving in the Air Force in Grand Forks, North Dakota from 1966 to 1968. It was there that his medical practice expanded to include hypnosis. Gene explored numerous other alternative therapies while practicing general medicine and general surgery at Williams Clinic in Ishpeming, Michigan from 1969 to 1987 and at the Thumb Butte Clinic in Prescott, Arizona from 1987 to 1996. Today, his specialties include hypnosis, chelation, oxidative medicine, Reiki, aromatherapy, prolotherapy, neurotherapy, thought field therapy, nutrition, homeopathy and kinesiology.

In 1997, Gene became a staff physician at the well-known Gerson Cancer Clinic in Sedona, Arizona. He also served as Chief of Staff at Bell Memorial Hospital in 1974 and is presently a board member at the Whole Child Resource Center in Prescott, Arizona, as well as an affiliate faculty member in Division Clinical Education at Midwestern University in Phoenix, Arizona.

Gene is a current member of the American Preventative Medicine Association and the Arizona Homeopathic Medicine Association. He is also a past member of the Arizona Medical Association, the American Medical Association and the Complementary Medicine Association of Arizona. Organizatios where Gene has served as a board member include the Complementary Medicine Association and Upper Peninsula Quality Assurance as well as the Audit Committee at Bell Memorial Hospital, where he served as board chairman.

Gene has also been a Medical Peer Review Committee member at Northern Michigan Review Association and a utilization review physician at the Acocks Medical Facility and the Mather Nursing Home. In addition, he has been a member as well as secretary of theUpper Peninsula Quality Assurance Information Analysis Committee, an advisory committee member at Upper Peninsula Home Nursing and a member of the Northern Michigan Corporation for Medical Care.

Index

C

G

V

Valerian root, 51
Valedictorian, 3
Vanadium, 26, 61, 80
Vasodilator, 63-64
Vegetable juice, 38-39
Vericose veins, 48
Veterinarian, 145
Vibrational medicine, 131
Vicks Vapor Rub, 22
Viral infections, 28, 48, 50, 127-128
Virgin olive oil, 36
Viruses, 33, 52, 123, 152
Visualization, 153
Vitamin A, 45, 118, 153
Vitamin B12, 44
Vitamin B6, 44, 48
Vitamin C, 18, 26-28, 42, 44-45, 48, 78, 107-108, 118, 153, 155, 179
Vitamin E, 26-27, 42-45, 47, 56, 58, 108, 124, 154
Vitamin K, 78
Voltaire, 30

W

Warts, 22
Water, 32-35, 40-41, 50, 65, 77, 81, 85-86, 96, 101, 117, 125-126, 128-129, 131, 141, 146, 154, 161-162, 166
Water of Life, The, 146
Water purifiers, 33
Waterborne disease, 33
Watermelon, 54
Weil, Dr. Andrew, 165
West Yellowstone, 11, 42
West, Dr. Bruce, 9, 40, 105
Wheat flour, 36
Wheezing, 66
Whey protein, 40
Whiplash, 143
Whiskey, 39

0-595-32580-7

Printed in the United States
23995LVS00004B/159

9 780595 325801